Home Portable Monitoring for Obstructive Sleep Apnea

Guest Editor

MICHAEL R. LITTNER, MD

SLEEP MEDICINE CLINICS

www.sleep.theclinics.com

September 2011 • Volume 6 • Number 3

SAUNDERS an imprint of ELSEVIER, Inc.

W.B. SAUNDERS COMPANY
A Division of Elsevier Inc.

1600 John F. Kennedy Boulevard • Suite 1800 • Philadelphia, PA 19103-2899

http://www.sleep.theclinics.com

SLEEP MEDICINE CLINICS Volume 6, Number 3
September 2011, ISSN 1556-407X, ISBN-13: 978-1-4557-1153-6

Editor: Sarah E. Barth
Developmental Editor: Donald E. Mumford

Sleep Medicine Clinics (ISSN 1556-407X) is published quarterly by Elsevier Inc., 360 Park Avenue South, New York, NY 10010-1710. Months of issue are March, June, September and December. Business and Editorial Offices: 1600 John F. Kennedy Blvd., Ste. 1800, Philadelphia, PA 19103-2899. Customer Service Office: 3251 Riverport Lane, Maryland Heights, MO 63043. Periodicals postage paid at New York, NY and additional mailing offices. Subscription prices are $161.00 per year (US individuals), $80.00 (US residents), $346.00 (US institutions), $198.00 (foreign individuals), $111.00 (foreign residents), and $381.00 (foreign institutions). Foreign air speed delivery is included in all *Clinics* subscription prices. All prices are subject to change without notice. **POSTMASTER:** Send change of address to *Sleep Medicine Clinics*, Elsevier Health Sciences Division, Subscription Customer Service, 3251 Riverport Lane, Maryland Heights, MO 63043. Customer Service: **Tel: 1-800-654-2452 (U.S. and Canada); 314-447-8871 (outside U.S. and Canada). Fax: 314-447-8029. E-mail: journalscustomerservice-usa@elsevier.com (for print support); journalsonlinesupport-usa@elsevier.com (for online support).**

Reprints. For copies of 100 or more of articles in this publication, please contact the Commercial Reprints Department, Elsevier Inc., 360 Park Avenue South, New York, NY 10010-1710. Tel.: 212-633-3812; Fax: 212-462-1935; E-mail: reprints@elsevier.com.

Printed and bound by CPI Group (UK) Ltd, Croydon, CR0 4YY

Transferred to Digital Print 2012

GOAL STATEMENT

The goal of *Sleep Clinics of North America* is to keep practicing physicians up to date with current clinical practice by providing timely articles reviewing the state of the art in patient care.

ACCREDITATION

The *Sleep Clinics of North America* is planned and implemented in accordance with the Essential Areas and Policies of the Accreditation Council for Continuing Medical Education (ACCME) through the joint sponsorship of the University of Virginia School of Medicine and Elsevier. The University of Virginia School of Medicine is accredited by the ACCME to provide continuing medical education for physicians.

The University of Virginia School of Medicine designates this enduring material activity for a maximum of 15 *AMA PRA Category 1 Credit*(s)™ for each issue, 60 credits per year. Physicians should only claim credit commensurate with the extent of their participation in the activity.

The American Medical Association has determined that physicians not licensed in the US who participate in this CME enduring material activity are eligible for a maximum of 15 *AMA PRA Category 1 Credit*(s)™ for each issue, 60 credits per year.

Credit can be earned by reading the text material, taking the CME examination online at http://www.theclinics.com/home/cme, and completing the evaluation. After taking the test, you will be required to review any and all incorrect answers. Following completion of the test and evaluation, your credit will be awarded and you may print your certificate.

FACULTY DISCLOSURE/CONFLICT OF INTEREST

The University of Virginia School of Medicine, as an ACCME accredited provider, endorses and strives to comply with the Accreditation Council for Continuing Medical Education (ACCME) Standards of Commercial Support, Commonwealth of Virginia statutes, University of Virginia policies and procedures, and associated federal and private regulations and guidelines on the need for disclosure and monitoring of proprietary and financial interests that may affect the scientific integrity and balance of content delivered in continuing medical education activities under our auspices.

The University of Virginia School of Medicine requires that all CME activities accredited through this institution be developed independently and be scientifically rigorous, balanced and objective in the presentation/discussion of its content, theories and practices.

All authors/editors participating in an accredited CME activity are expected to disclose to the readers relevant financial relationships with commercial entities occurring within the past 12 months (such as grants or research support, employee, consultant, stock holder, member of speakers bureau, etc.). The University of Virginia School of Medicine will employ appropriate mechanisms to resolve potential conflicts of interest to maintain the standards of fair and balanced education to the reader. Questions about specific strategies can be directed to the Office of Continuing Medical Education, University of Virginia School of Medicine, Charlottesville, Virginia.

The faculty and staff of the University of Virginia Office of Continuing Medical Education have no financial affiliations to disclose.

The authors/editors listed below have identified no professional or financial affiliations for themselves or their spouse/partner:
Dennis R. Bailey, DDS; Sarah Barth (Acquisitions Editor); Cynthia Brown, MD (Test Author); Nancy Collop, MD; Shilpa Guggali, MD; Sean Hesselbacher, MD; Amarbir Mattewal, MD; Kavita Mundey, MD; Carol L. Rosen, MD; and Parina Shah, MD.

The authors/editors listed below identified the following professional or financial affiliations for themselves or their spouse/partner:
Richard B. Berry, MD is an industry funded research/investigator for Ventus Medical and Philips-Respironics.
Indira Gurubhagavatula, MD, MPH is the principal for screening for obstructive sleep apnea for Embla, Inc.
Max Hirshkowitz, PhD is on the Speakers' Bureau for Somaxon and Cephalon.
Samuel T. Kuna, MD is employed and industry funded by Philips Respironics.
Teofilo Lee-Chiong Jr, MD (Consulting Editor) is an industry funded research/investigator for Respironics and Embla.
Michael R. Littner, MD (Guest Editor) is a consultant for Balboa Sleep Disorders Laboratory, and is on the Speakers' Bureau for the Journal of Clinical Sleep Medicine and Sleep (a medical Journal, AASM & SRS).
Amir Sharafkhaneh, MD, PhD is a consultant, is on the Speakers' Bureau, and is on the Advisory Committee/Board for GSK, BI, Pfizer, and DEY.
Philip R. Westbrook, MD is employed, industry funded, consultant, on the advisory committee/board, owns stock and patent holder for Advanced Brain Monitoring, Inc. Also employed, consultant and owns stock In Watermark Medical, LLC and Ventus Medical, Inc. Employed and consultant for Rotech, Inc.
B. Tucker Woodson, MD is a consultant for Medtronic and Inspire Medical, receives royalty from Medtronic ENT, and is an industry funded research/investigator for Inspire Medical.

Disclosure of Discussion of Non-FDA Approved Uses for Pharmaceutical Products and/or Medical Devices
The University of Virginia School of Medicine, as an ACCME provider, requires that all faculty presenters identify and disclose any off-label uses for pharmaceutical and medical device products. The University of Virginia School of Medicine recommends that each physician fully review all the available data on new products or procedures prior to clinical use.

TO ENROLL

To enroll in the Sleep Clinics of North America Continuing Medical Education program, call customer service at 1-800-654-2452 or visit us online at www.theclinics.com/home/cme. The CME program is available to subscribers for an additional fee of $114.00.

Sleep Medicine Clinics

THE CLINICS ARE NOW AVAILABLE ONLINE!

Access your subscription at:
www.theclinics.com

Contributors

CONSULTING EDITOR

TEOFILO LEE-CHIONG Jr, MD

Professor of Medicine and Chief, Division of Sleep Medicine, National Jewish Health; Associate Professor of Medicine, University of Colorado Denver School of Medicine, Denver, Colorado

GUEST EDITOR

MICHAEL R. LITTNER, MD

Emeritus Professor of Medicine, David Geffen School of Medicine at University of California, Los Angeles, Los Angeles, California

AUTHORS

DENNIS R. BAILEY, DDS

Visiting Lecturer in Orofacial Pain and Dental Sleep Medicine Department; Co-Director, Dental Sleep Mini-Residency, University of California Los Angeles School of Dentistry, Los Angeles, California

RICHARD B. BERRY, MD

Professor of Medicine; Medical Director, UF & Shands Sleep Disorders Center; Division of Pulmonary, Critical Care, and Sleep Medicine, University of Florida, Gainesville, Florida

NANCY COLLOP, MD

Professor of Medicine, Emory University, Atlanta, Georgia

SHILPA GUGGALI, MD

Resident, Department of Psychiatry and Behavioral Medicine, The Medical College of Wisconsin, Milwaukee, Wisconsin

INDIRA GURUBHAGAVATULA, MD, MPH

Division of Sleep Medicine, University of Pennsylvania; Pulmonary, Critical Care and Sleep Section, Philadelphia Veterans Affairs Medical Center, Sleep Center, Philadelphia, Pennsylvania

SEAN HESSELBACHER, MD

Pulmonary, Critical Care and Sleep Medicine Section, Department of Medicine, Baylor College of Medicine, Houston, Texas

MAX HIRSHKOWITZ, PhD

Associate Professor of Medicine and Psychiatry, Section Pulmonary, Critical Care and Sleep Medicine, Department of Medicine and Menninger Department of Psychiatry, Baylor College of Medicine; Director, Sleep Disorders & Research Center, Section of Pulmonary, Critical Care and Sleep Medicine, Medical Care Line, Michael E. DeBakey VA Medical Center, Houston, Texas

SAMUEL T. KUNA, MD

Chief, Pulmonary, Critical Care and Sleep Medicine, Philadelphia Veterans Affairs Medical Center; Associate Professor of Medicine, University of Pennsylvania School of Medicine, Philadelphia, Pennsylvania

AMARBIR MATTEWAL, MD

Pulmonary, Critical Care and Sleep Medicine Section, Department of Medicine, Baylor College of Medicine, Houston, Texas

KAVITA MUNDEY, MD
Assistant Professor, Division of Pulmonary, Critical Care and Sleep Medicine, Medical College of Wisconsin; Director, Sleep Medicine Program, Clement J. Zablocki Veterans Affairs Medical Center, Milwaukee, Wisconsin

CAROL L. ROSEN, MD
Professor, Department of Pediatrics, Division of Pediatric Pulmonary, Allergy and Immunology, and Sleep Medicine, Case Western Reserve University School of Medicine; Medical Director, Pediatric Sleep Center, Rainbow Babies and Children's Hospital, University Hospitals Case Medical Center, Cleveland, Ohio

PARINA SHAH, MD
Division of Sleep Medicine, University of Pennsylvania, Philadelphia, Pennsylvania

AMIR SHARAFKHANEH, MD, PhD
Associate Professor of Medicine & Program Director, Sleep Medicine Fellowship Program, Section Pulmonary, Critical Care and Sleep Medicine, Department of Medicine, Baylor College of Medicine; Medical Director, Sleep Disorders & Research Center, Section of Pulmonary, Critical Care and Sleep Medicine, Medical Care Line, Michael E. DeBakey VA Medical Center, Houston, Texas

PHILIP R. WESTBROOK, MD
Emeritus Associate Professor of Medicine, Mayo Clinic College of Medicine, Rochester, Minnesota; Emeritus Clinical Professor of Medicine, David Geffen School of Medicine, University of California Los Angeles, Los Angeles; Chief Medical Officer, Advanced Brain Monitoring, Inc., Carlsbad, California; Chief Medical Officer, Watermark Medical, Inc., Florida; Chief Medical Officer, Ventus Medical, Inc., California

B. TUCKER WOODSON, MD
Professor, Department of Otolaryngology and Communication Sciences; Chief, Division of Sleep Medicine, Medical College of Wisconsin, Milwaukee, Wisconsin

Contents

> Obstructive sleep apnea is a prevalent disease associated with increased morbidity and mortality. As awareness about the disorder grows, the number of sleep laboratory referrals increases tremendously, along with health care costs. Furthermore, in health care systems with fixed budgets, long waiting times delay diagnosis and therapy. To overcome some difficulties and expedite delivery of care, unattended portable monitoring devices greatly interest practitioners, sleep centers, and third-party payors for diagnosing sleep-disordered breathing. This article reviews the technical aspects and options available for portable home testing of sleep apnea.

> Cardiopulmonary home sleep testing (HST) devices are tools of verification for diagnosing sleep-related breathing disorders. They can rule-in but not rule-out diagnosis. Types, channels, capabilities, and validation vary widely. Overall recording technique, scoring practices, the types of problems encountered, and interpretation strategies for cardiopulmonary recorders differ greatly from those used in traditional sleep studies. Diagnostic sensitivity with HST is lower than that for polysomnography, largely due to data limitations. Nonetheless, the shortcomings are usually offset by performing home sleep tests only on patients with high pretest probabilities for sleep-disordered breathing.

> Portable monitors for home unattended testing of patients with obstructive sleep apnea are gaining increasing acceptance. Portable monitors vary widely in the signals recorded and must be interpreted with knowledge of their performance capabilities. Comparison of results on portable monitor testing and polysomnography depend on differences in technology, testing location, and night-to-night variability of sleep apnea severity. Recent comparative effectiveness research is comparing the clinical outcomes after in-laboratory versus home portable monitor testing to determine how these monitors should best be applied to clinical medicine.

obstructive sleep apnea, the high expense of in-laboratory sleep studies, the current economic environment, and the rapid pace of technological advancements have all contributed toward the increased use of portable sleep monitoring for the diagnosis of obstructive sleep apnea. This article reviews important aspects of portable sleep monitoring and provides clinical examples to aid the practitioner in the application of this rapidly evolving technology.

Diagnostic testing for obstructive sleep apnea is moving into a new era in which many patients will be tested in their homes rather than in the sleep centers. Physicians performing such testing should be versed in the practice of sleep medicine so that they can appropriately choose which patients can be accurately diagnosed with such testing; understand the types of devices; how to perform, score, and interpret these tests; and recommend treatment options. They must develop algorithms for such testing that include what to do with negative tests (true or false negatives), inadequate tests, or unexpected results.

This article explores some of the questions surrounding portable recording in the diagnosis and management of sleep-disordered breathing and what future research might be required to answer these questions. Evidence that the polysomnograph remains necessary for the routine clinical diagnosis of sleep-disordered breathing is discussed. Posited is a hypothetical portable device that meets the spirit if not quite all the letters of the AASM recommendations for portable recording technology. The term "value," meaning health outcomes per dollar spent, is used in addressing research needs. Achieving high value in health care is what is "in the best interest of the patient."

Foreword

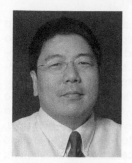

Teofilo Lee-Chiong Jr, MD
Consulting Editor

Home sleep testing (HST)—are we ready for it? In order to understand some of the concerns raised about HST, and to determine how this diagnostic tool was being utilized across the nation, a survey of nearly a hundred leading authorities in home sleep testing was conducted—these included clinicians, researchers, sleep center managers, and device manufacturers. Each one was asked to respond to these ten questions:

1. Why should centers *without* existing in-laboratory polysomnography (PSG) sleep programs start a HST program? Or should they not start one?
2. Why should centers *with* existing PSG programs start a HST program? Or should they not start one?
3. What are the potential *advantages* of HST over a PSG program?
4. What are the potential *disadvantages* of HST compared to a PSG program? What are the possible *adverse consequences* of starting a HST program?
5. What are the *factors* that need to be considered in starting a HST program?
6. What are the *resources* needed to start a HST program?
7. What are the factors that should be considered when choosing a specific HST *device*?
8. What factors would you consider in choosing a *staff* for the HST program? Any special qualifications? Job descriptions?
9. What type of *patients* would be appropriate for HST? What type of patients would be inappropriate for HST? What information would be needed for the patient intake?
10. How would you assess an HST program's *performance*?

Replies ranged from optimism to concern, were broad-ranging or limited in scope to a specific sleep medicine center, and were either philosophical or practical, or both.

WHY SHOULD CENTERS *WITHOUT* EXISTING IN-LABORATORY PSG SLEEP PROGRAMS START A HST PROGRAM? OR SHOULD THEY NOT START ONE?

To enable quicker access was a common response, as well as providing better, more comprehensive patient care to ensure better patient outcomes, to increase direct clinic revenue, and to manage patient care expenses. Some respondents, however, cautioned against starting a HST program in any facility that does not have an in-laboratory PSG program to repeat tests that were of insufficient quality, that do not otherwise provide a clear diagnosis, or that showed negative results in persons highly suspected of having sleep-disordered breathing. An in-laboratory PSG program is also crucial for positive airway pressure (PAP) titration studies and for evaluating patients with low pretest probability for sleep apnea but with high pretest probability for other sleep disorders.

WHY SHOULD CENTERS *WITH* EXISTING PSG PROGRAMS START A HST PROGRAM? OR SHOULD THEY NOT START ONE?

Again, many reasons were provided: to accommodate demand and increase access to patients; to increase the number of patients currently diagnosed and treated for obstructive sleep apnea (OSA); to increase clinical revenue; to reduce expenses for patients who cannot afford an in-laboratory sleep study; and to provide follow-up

Sleep Med Clin 6 (2011) xi–xiii
doi:10.1016/j.jsmc.2011.06.001

evaluation for patients with OSA, especially those who have chosen oral devices or upper airway surgery as therapy for their condition, or those with suboptimal response to PAP treatment. Many see some potential for marketing (ie, to compete with other sleep medicine centers in the community in the provision of care), while others believe that it is inevitable that some insurance carriers will force HST before approving in-laboratory PSG.

WHAT ARE THE POTENTIAL ADVANTAGES OF HST OVER A PSG PROGRAM?

Numerous advantages were mentioned, including testing in a more natural sleeping environment, lower capital resources to program building, less cost to insurance carriers and patients, greater (easier) access/convenience for patients, reduction in wait time, and ease of interpretation by both sleep technologists and clinicians.

WHAT ARE THE POTENTIAL DISADVANTAGES OF HST COMPARED TO A PSG PROGRAM? WHAT ARE THE POSSIBLE ADVERSE CONSEQUENCES OF STARTING A HST PROGRAM?

Some are concerned about the lower quality of studies and less accurate results; lack of sleep technologist observation and, if needed, intervention; lack of data regarding sleep architecture and periodic limb movements (to name just a few); more uncertainty with borderline studies and greater amount of uninterpretable studies; and the difficulty in differentiating disorders other than OSA leading to less attention to non-OSA sleep disorders. It is commonly held that, as a screening tool, HST is not cost-effective, and as a stand-alone diagnostic modality, HST is unreliable—that false-positive studies may lead to unnecessary or inappropriate treatment, whereas ambiguous results may delay treatment. Finally, it had been argued that wide adoption of HST will have an adverse economic impact on many, if not most, sleep centers, while, at the same time, it may lead to overuse or abuse, with HST being ordered indiscriminately.

WHAT ARE THE FACTORS THAT NEED TO BE CONSIDERED IN STARTING A HST PROGRAM?

There is agreement that access to support in the middle of the night if needed is indispensable, as are accessibility of in-laboratory PSG services and to sleep medicine specialists.

WHAT ARE THE RESOURCES NEEDED TO START A HST PROGRAM?

First and foremost is education, not only for sleep medicine clinicians and sleep technologists, but also for referring physicians and other health care providers, insurance carriers, durable medical equipment suppliers, and patients and their families.

Other crucial resources are adequate staffing to screen potential patients, to educate on how to conduct the testing, review and score test data, to clean equipment prior to reuse, and to provide follow-up care; office space, which, at a minimum, should include an education room/setup area, storage room, and a reading station; and an adequate number of HST devices, including back-up devices in case of loss/nonreturns or damage to the equipment.

WHAT ARE THE FACTORS THAT SHOULD BE CONSIDERED WHEN CHOOSING A SPECIFIC HST DEVICE?

This was easy—it was almost universally agreed upon that devices should demonstrate reliability and high validity; be accurate when compared to the gold-standard, the in-laboratory PSG; provide high-quality data (eg, how are artifacts controlled); be easy to download and store data, and easy to use by both patient and sleep staff; allow full disclosure of raw data (ie, it should not be a "black box"); be able to synchronize with "smart" PAP devices; permit determination of sleep position; be relatively durable but inexpensive (including consumable supplies); be able to monitor over several nights; be able to identify problems and provide solutions to problems; be able to allow patients to determine if acceptable data were collected prior to returning the HST device to the sleep center; have the ability to manually score raw data; and, ideally, be compatible to existing in-laboratory PSG equipment.

WHAT FACTORS WOULD YOU CONSIDER IN CHOOSING A STAFF FOR THE HST PROGRAM? ANY SPECIAL QUALIFICATIONS? JOB DESCRIPTIONS?

This was more difficult—respondents provided conflicting expectations and job descriptions. One camp believed in using only experienced registered sleep technologists, while the opposite group felt that applying limited-channel HST devices is fairly straightforward and does not require special training in the use and interpretation of PSGs.

WHAT TYPE OF PATIENTS WOULD BE APPROPRIATE FOR HST? WHAT TYPE OF PATIENTS WOULD BE INAPPROPRIATE FOR HST? WHAT INFORMATION WOULD BE NEEDED FOR THE PATIENT INTAKE?

This issue will continue to be debated as technology improves, and as sleep staff acquires more experience with HST protocols. For now, it is commonly accepted that patients who are possibly appropriate for HST include those with clear, uncomplicated OSA or those with high likelihood of OSA. Possibly inappropriate are more complicated cases including patients with multisystemic disorders, non-OSA sleep disorders, heart failure, obesity hypoventilation syndrome, nocturnal seizures or complex parasomnias, as well as patients who are overly anxious about home testing or who are uncomfortable with technology (eg, someone like me). At this time, children are not appropriate candidates for HST.

HOW WOULD YOU ASSESS A HST?

Responses included the following: quality of data; turn-around time for reports; reach—geographically and economically; frequency of equipment failure or need for repeat HST or in-laboratory PSG; patient satisfaction; referring physician satisfaction; treatment compliance.

Home sleep testing—are we ready for it? The questions are not "Why?" but rather "Why not?," "When?," and How?"

Teofilo Lee-Chiong Jr, MD
Division of Sleep Medicine
National Jewish Health
University of Colorado Denver School of Medicine
1400 Jackson Street, Room J221
Denver, CO 60206, USA

E-mail address:
Lee-ChiongT@NJC.ORG

Preface

Portable Monitors for Home Sleep Testing for the Diagnosis and Follow-up of Obstructive Sleep Apnea: Past, Present, and Future

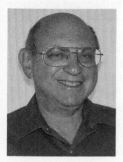

Michael R. Littner, MD
Guest Editor

This issue of *Sleep Medicine Clinics* examines the use of portable monitors (PM) for unattended, home testing for the diagnosis of obstructive sleep apnea (OSA). The articles review our current understanding of the role of PMs in adults and children. The first 4 topics cover technical aspects of PMs, scoring strategies, outcome measures to assess the long-term efficacy, and how to integrate PMs into an overall clinical program. The next 3 topics examine the use in patients for whom there is little information at this time to guide clinical practice. These are patients for whom a dental appliance or upper airway surgery is being considered, and pediatric patients. The last 3 topics review practical aspects of the use of PMs with examples of PM recordings, a review of current published standards for the use of PMs, and what needs to be done in the future to better understand the role of PMs.

There is a long history of PMs for unattended testing. Although home sleep testing (HST) dates at least to 1981,[1] perhaps the most important advance was the introduction of relatively inexpensive pulse oximeters for portable measurement of arterial hemoglobin saturation plus the ability to save the information for subsequent review and interpretation. Some of the earliest approaches involved the use of oximetry alone

but more complex commercial systems followed quickly. It soon became apparent that the use of PMs was based on a number of factors such as ease of access and cost compared to full, in-laboratory, attended polysomnography (PSG). It may be argued that the popularity of split-night PSG,[2] in which the first portion of the night provides a diagnosis and the second half of the night provides a opportunity for positive airway pressure (PAP) titration, was a result, at least in part, of the advent of PMs. The split-night approach makes the PSG potentially more cost-effective compared to PMs since it may eliminate a second night of PSG for PAP titration. However, despite the potential for use of PMs, there was scant evidence to guide practitioners and the American Academy of Sleep Medicine (AASM) (then known as the American Sleep Disorders Association) convened a task force to evaluate evidence for the use of PMs. The task force and subsequent practice parameters did not generally support the use of PMs based on the evidence. However, the task force developed a classification system (well described in several of the articles in this issue) that has become the basis for virtually all subsequent reviews of PMs.

Subsequent to the publication of the 1994 practice parameters on PMs, a number of studies were

Sleep Med Clin 6 (2011) xv–xvii
doi:10.1016/j.jsmc.2011.05.013
1556-407X/11/$ – see front matter

performed and several evidence-based reviews up to 2004 were conducted as outlined in Dr Collop's article. Each of these reviews concluded that the use of PMs for unattended HST could not be supported by the evidence when compared to PSG. However, a joint review by the AASM, American Thoracic Society, and American College of Chest Physicians[3] provided a framework for subsequent study designs and indicated that patient-centered outcomes in addition to the apnea/hypopnea index (AHI) from HST compared to PSG would be appropriate and even preferred measures. Specifically, the review stated, "Another useful approach will be to assess diagnosis and management strategies with decision branches that include both polysomnography and portable monitoring. Each strategy could be investigated to determine whether outcomes such as symptoms, health status, health-care utilization, or cost-effectiveness are comparable for each branch of a given algorithm and could be considered a validation of a clinical practice guideline." There have now been several studies published or in process that have used this approach with the addition of PAP treatment as part of the management strategy and PAP acceptance and adherence as part of the outcomes. These are reviewed by Dr Berry, Dr Kuna, and Dr Collop in this issue. Of note, the use of positive pressure in sleep disorders including the use of continuous PAP, auto-titrating PAP (APAP), and other modalities of PAP have been covered in another issue of *Sleep Medicine Clinics*.[4] In addition, PAP and APAP are the subject of practice parameters by the AASM.[5,6]

After the joint review, the AASM produced a set of clinical guidelines for the use of PMs in 2007. Between 2008 and 2009, the Center for Medicare and Medicaid Services conducted further reviews as outlined by Dr Berry and Dr Collop. Based, in part, on expert panel recommendations, the Center for Medicare and Medicaid Services approved the use of PMs that had at least 3 recording channels, 1 of which must be a measure (directly or indirectly) of airflow for use to qualify patients for PAP therapy.

More recently (January 2011), the AASM has adopted accreditation standards for out-of-center testing for OSA as outlined in Dr Collop's article. Thus, the evolution of HST using PMs has gone from a concept to practical equipment to evidence-based support to a reimbursable test to currently a potentially major component of the approach to diagnosis of OSA. Further, the approach is supported by clinical guidelines[7] and an accreditation process from the AASM.

However, substantial barriers still remain to both implement PM diagnostic approaches and provide quality patient care. The large number of PMs commercially available, as outlined in Dr Hesselbacher's article (44 listed in Table 2), indicates the current mainstream use of PMs. However, it also highlights the difficulty a practitioner has in determining which device is most appropriate in the practitioner's clinical setting. In addition, almost all studies with the use of PMs focused on high-risk patients, generally those who had an AHI greater than 15 hours of sleep. In these patients, acceptance and adherence were similar to what is expected when using PSG to diagnose and guide subsequent PAP treatment (reviews by Dr Berry and Dr Kuna in this issue). However, in 1 study that examined patients with mild OSA, acceptance and adherence were extremely low with only 3 of 69 patients with an AHI <10 on a HST being compliant at 3 months.[8] In addition, in those studies that enrolled high-risk patients without comorbidities and reported the number of patients who failed to qualify, only a small minority of patients were suitable for use of PMs (as reviewed by Dr Berry in this issue). Scoring strategies are also in evolution, as reviewed in Dr Hirshkowitz's article. While patients with high-quality data from a PM and obvious OSA are easily diagnosed, data quality may not always be ideal but still interpretable. Dr Hirshkowitz has provided a recommendation to quantify the result by adjusting the AHI based on the quality of the data and then comparing the final result to a table of likelihoods that the patient has OSA. A decision can then be made to either proceed with treatment, repeat the study, or proceed to a PSG.

There is still a great deal of work to be done in better understanding which patients are suitable for PMs. The reviews of Dr Bailey on dental appliances, Dr Mundey on upper airway surgery, and Dr Rosen on pediatric patients all indicate that the use of portable monitoring for primary diagnosis and follow-up still requires study to better understand the role of PMs in these cases.

With each of the articles in this issue focusing on a particular subject area, integration of the information for patient care may be difficult. Dr Shah's article has provided guidance to evaluate patients for possible HST and examples of the type of recordings that are likely to be obtained and how to interpret these recordings.

Finally, Dr Westbrook has looked into his crystal ball and provided some projections on the future of the use of PMs.

Based on the articles in issue, PMs can be effective tools in the diagnostic approach to patients with symptoms and signs of OSA. However, as reviewed by Dr Berry and Dr Kuna, selection of patients is critical, treatment approaches must be carefully considered, and outcomes once the patient is treated need to be monitored closely. Nondiagnostic studies in high-risk patients need to be followed up carefully, often with a repeat HST or a PSG. Finally, as reviewed by Dr Collop, out-of-center use of PMs requires a coordinated effort by a well-trained staff who have met the high standards put forth by the AASM to ensure a high quality of patient care.

Michael R. Littner, MD
David Geffen School of Medicine
University of California, Los Angeles
Los Angeles, CA 90024, USA

E-mail address:
mlittner@ucla.edu

REFERENCES

1. Ancoli-Israel S, Kripke DF, Mason W, et al. Comparisons of home sleep recordings and polysomnograms in older adults with sleep disorders. Sleep 1981;4:283–91.
2. Iber C, O'Brien C, Schluter J, et al. Single night studies in obstructive sleep apnea. Sleep 1991;14:383–5.
3. Flemons WW, Littner MR, Rowley JA, et al. Home diagnosis of sleep apnea: a systematic review of the literature: an evidence review cosponsored by the American Academy of Sleep Medicine, the American College of Chest Physicians, and the American Thoracic Society. Chest 2003;124:1543–79.
4. Berry RB, editor. Positive airway pressure therapy. Sleep Med Clin 2010;5(3).
5. Kushida CA, Littner MR, Hirshkowitz M, et al. Practice parameters for the use of continuous and bilevel positive airway pressure devices to treat adult patients with sleep-related breathing disorders. Sleep 2006;29:375–80.
6. Morgenthaler TI, Aurora RN, Brown T, et al. Practice parameters for the use of autotitrating continuous positive airway pressure devices for titrating pressures and treating adult patients with obstructive sleep apnea syndrome: an update for 2007. An American Academy of Sleep Medicine report. Sleep 2008;31:141–7.
7. Collop N, Anderson M, Boehloecke B, et al. Clinical guidelines for the use of portable monitoring in adult patients. J Clin Sleep Med 2007;3:737–47.
8. Whitelaw WA, Brant RF, Flemons WW. Clinical usefulness of home oximetry compared with polysomnography for assessment of sleep apnea. Am J Respir Crit Care Med 2005;171:188–93.

Classification, Technical Specifications, and Types of Home Sleep Testing Devices for Sleep-Disordered Breathing

Sean Hesselbacher, MD[a,1], Amarbir Mattewal, MD[a,1], Max Hirshkowitz, PhD[b], Amir Sharafkhaneh, MD, PhD[b,*]

KEYWORDS

- Apnea • Hypopnea • Monitoring • Diagnosis

Obstructive sleep apnea (OSA) is a major public health problem, affecting up to 5% of the world population[1] and between 2% and 4% of adults in the United States.[2] It is characterized by periods of breathing cessation (apnea) and periods of reduced breathing (hypopnea). Both types of events have similar pathophysiology and consequences for patients.[3] The severity of the disorder is quantified by measuring the number of apneas and hypopneas per hour of sleep (ie, the apnea-hypopnea index [AHI]). The standard approach to diagnosis is in-laboratory, technician-attended polysomnography (PSG). PSG requires technical expertise, is labor-intensive, and is time-consuming. Timely access to diagnostic testing is a problem for many patients, delayed diagnosis is common, and the costs associated with conducting in-laboratory PSG remain high.[4] Therefore, alternative approaches to diagnosis, such as portable monitoring (PM), have been proposed as a substitute for PSG in the diagnostic assessment of patients with suspected sleep apnea. The term "portable monitoring" encompasses a wide range of devices that may record a single channel or as many signals as attended PSG. Usually, electroencephalogram (EEG) and electromyogram (EMG) signals required for sleep-versus-wake differentiation are not recorded by portable monitors. Consequently, breathing events must be indexed per hour of monitoring time rather than by sleep time. The Center for Medicare & Medicaid Services (CMS) calls this new parameter the "respiratory disturbance index" (RDI). However, this term has created confusion because it was already in use and is widely understood by sleep specialists to mean the number of apneas, hypopneas, and respiratory effort–related arousals per hour of sleep. Therefore, rather than add to the confusion created by CMS, this article refers to the new use of the term RDI as "RDI-MD" (RDI Medicare-defined).

PM devices have been used investigationally for diagnosing OSA for more than 3 decades. With the advancement in technology, they are now a more viable option for the diagnosis and management of OSA. The potential benefits of using these devices in clinical practice include early diagnosis,

[a] Pulmonary, Critical Care and Sleep Medicine Section, Department of Medicine, Baylor College of Medicine, Houston, TX, USA
[b] Michael E. DeBakey VA Medical Center, Sleep Disorders & Research Center, Building 100, Room 6C-344, 2002 Holcombe Boulevard, Houston, TX 77030, USA
[1] Both authors contributed equally.
* Corresponding author.
E-mail address: amirs@bcm.tmc.edu

Sleep Med Clin 6 (2011) 261–282
doi:10.1016/j.jsmc.2011.05.010
1556-407X/11/$ – see front matter. Published by Elsevier Inc.

quicker treatment of OSA, reduced costs, the comfort and convenience of sleeping in one's own bed, and possibly achieving a more representative night's sleep. However, home sleep testing (HST) has several limitations, including the inherent lack of an attendant during the study (which may adversely affect data quality) and inability to assess sleep architecture, arousals, or other sleep disturbances. Furthermore, the large number of devices, manufacturers, channel configurations, and scoring schemes result in variability. Most devices still lack adequate validation in large patient samples. Finally, long-term outcome for patients diagnosed using PM devices is unknown.

In 1994, the American Sleep Disorders Association (now the American Academy of Sleep Medicine [AASM]) published its initial practice parameters regarding the use of PM devices for assessing OSA.[5] The society classified sleep apnea evaluation studies based on the number of channels or signals on the monitor and categorized them from level I to level IV. In 1997, the AASM published practice parameters[6] and a review[7] regarding indications for PSG and related procedures that included a section on level II and level IV studies. Based on the review, the practice parameters recommended that attended level III studies were potentially appropriate in patients with a high pretest probability (eg, >70%) for sleep apnea. Subsequently, an increasing amount of research has been published on PM for diagnosing sleep apnea.

In 2007, the AASM released the clinical guidelines for the use of unattended portable monitors in the diagnosis of OSA in adult patients.[8] The taskforce recommendations included the following: (1) PM for suspected OSA should be performed only in conjunction with a comprehensive sleep evaluation; (2) PM may be used as an alternative to PSG only in patients with a high pretest probability of moderate to severe OSA; (3) PM should not be used in patients with comorbid medical conditions or in whom comorbid sleep disorders are suspected; (4) a PM must record airflow, respiratory effort, and blood oxygenation; (5) an experienced sleep technologist should apply the PM sensors or directly educate the patient about the correct application; (6) methodology should be available to monitor the quality of recordings; (7) PM devices must display the raw data; and (8) all patients undergoing PM should have a follow-up visit to discuss the results of the test.

CMS has approved some PMs for diagnosing OSA and initiating CPAP.[9] The PMs that are considered acceptable include levels II and III. Some confusion existed regarding the use of level IV portable monitors, because CMS redefined a level IV monitor as one that uses three channels, one of which includes a measure of airflow (https://www.cms.gov/transmittals/downloads/R96NCD.pdf).

This remainder of this article discusses the technical aspects and options available for portable home testing devices for diagnosing sleep apnea.

CLASSIFICATION OF MONITORING DEVICES

Level I monitoring consists of full overnight PSG, with a minimum of two channels each for EEG, chin EMG, electrooculogram (EOG), respiratory airflow (with a thermistor or pressure-flow transducer), respiratory effort (thoracic and abdominal breathing movements), oximetry, and ECG or heart rate monitoring (**Table 1**). These studies are fully attended by a technologist and are typically conducted in a sleep center. These studies are not discussed in this article.

Level II PMs consist of an equivalent number of channels as level I, but the study is not attended by a technician. Level II recordings require setup by a trained technologist. Level II studies allow for the identification and quantification of sleep stages; calculation of total sleep time; recognition of arousals; and scoring of leg movements. These data, in turn, permit determination of stage-specific OSA severity, and recognition of cause-and-effect relationships among respiratory abnormalities, leg movements, and arousals. These data also enable clinicians to exclude waking respiratory irregularities from summary calculations. However, the computerized sleep-staging settings installed by the manufacturers vary among devices. Nonetheless, the devices' sensitivity and specificity for diagnosing OSA reached 100% and 93%, respectively, in one study.[10]

Level III monitors record a minimum of four channels that must include oximetry, one or more channels of respiratory effort or movement, heart rate, and a measure of airflow. Level III devices are relatively simple to use, and patients are able to apply the sensors themselves to perform their recordings at home. These devices do not record EEG, EOG, or chin EMG, and therefore do not allow for direct determination of wakefulness and the stages of sleep. With these monitoring devices, calculating what is traditionally called RDI is not possible, and RDI-MD potentially underestimates severity if a patient is awake for a significant part of the study. Data loss (reported loss of 4%–24%) is another major problem with level III portable devices.[11–13]

Level IV monitors record only one or two channels, typically including oxygen saturation or airflow. Some other signals that have been studied

Table 1
American Academy of Sleep Medicine classification of levels of studies of sleep apnea evaluation

	Level 1	Level 2	Level 3	Level 4
Description	Standard attended PSG	Comprehensive portable PSG	Modified portable sleep apnea testing	Continuous single or dual bioparameter recording
Measures	Minimum of seven, including EEG, EOG, chin EMG, ECG, airflow, respiratory effort, oxygen saturation	Minimum of seven, including EEG, EOG, chin EMG, ECG or heart rate, airflow, respiratory effort, oxygen saturation	Minimum of four, including ventilation (at least two channels of respiratory movement, or respiratory movement and airflow), heart rate or ECG, oxygen saturation	Minimum of one: oxygen saturation, flow, or chest movement
Body position	Documented or objectively measured	May be objectively measured	May be objectively measured	Not measured
Leg movement	EMG or motion sensor desirable but optional	EMG or motion sensor desirable but optional	May be recorded	Not recorded
Personnel	In constant attendance	Not in attendance	Not in attendance	Not in attendance
Interventions	Possible	Not possible	Not possible	Not possible

Abbreviations: ECG, electrocardiography; EEG, electroencephalography; EMG, electromyography; EOG, electrooculography; PSG, polysomnography.
Data from Ferber R, Millman R, Coppola M, et al. Portable recording in the assessment of obstructive sleep apnea. Sleep 1994;17(4):378–92.

include ECG, heart rate, blood pressure, and body movement. Recently, the Agency for Healthcare Research and Quality (AHRQ) broadened the definition of level IV monitors to include all devices not meeting criteria for level III devices.[14] The data from these devices combined with a pretest clinical score can increase the sensitivity, and may be useful in screening.

Novel technologies in PM have also been developed and marketed, incorporating unconventional signals (eg, peripheral arterial tonometry and actigraphy) and different combinations of signals that do not match the traditional AASM classification categories.[15,16] Overall, commercially available PMs lack standardization. The monitors, even those within the same class, are not equivalent, and no studies have compared different PM devices head-to-head. Furthermore, what combination of signals produces the best diagnostic sensitivity and specificity is unknown.[8]

TECHNOLOGIES USED IN INDIVIDUAL PM DEVICES

The type of technology, or combination of technologies, used in an individual PM device plays a significant role in the size of the device, ease of application, and interpretability of the data. It also has financial implications to the provider. Devices vary widely in the amount of information provided and complexity, and therefore the primary factor in choosing a device is the type of information needed from the study. **Table 2** provides a summary of the technical specifications of the individual devices currently available in the United States.

An important consideration is that these studies are meant to be performed at home, in an uncontrolled environment. Each additional lead used in a device increases the opportunity for data loss during the night, but may also provide redundancy. Thus, a single missing lead may not be as important to the final clinical interpretation. The Sleep Heart Health Study,[29–33] using the PS-2 (Compumedics) level II device, found that 91% of the 6802 initial home studies were acceptable. The study also showed that obese patients had a lower likelihood of successful initial study. The oximeter probe was the sensor that provided adequate data for the largest proportion in the study (93% of the average study duration), followed by EOG, EEG, chin, chest, thermocouple, and, finally, the abdominal sensor. Although some aspects of individual devices are highlighted here, the combination of features provided by each device is unique and are listed in **Table 3**.

Level II Devices

Most of the PM devices currently on the market are simplifications of technologies used in standard laboratory PSG. Level II devices are intended to perform similarly to level I devices, except that they are used in an unattended setting. Many devices are marketed as both level I and II recorders. These tests are appropriate when sleep state is important or electroencephalographic abnormalities during sleep are suspected. Some tests can also be used for ambulatory EEG recording. Attempts to solve EEG lead malfunction problems during the night have produced innovations, such as digital filtering and mechanical devices like the 10/20 BraiNet Template (Cadwell, Kennewick, WA, USA). Other devices limit EEG recording to one to two channels that may simplify setup while providing data about sleep state. More data channels may shorten battery life or fill available data storage, shortening recording time. Because many level II devices require setup by a technologist (which may occur during the day of the intended sleep test), features intended to delay recording initiation include timers that can be set to start recording near bedtime, a button that can serve as an event recorder, or a start/stop button for the patient to push at bed/wake times. Techniques developed to allow remote monitoring of home studies include using wireless/cellular technology from the DreamPort. This device uses a wireless receiver and transmitter designed for the Crystal Monitor and Sapphire PSG systems (CleveMed, Cleveland, OH, USA).[21–28] Other options include modem/Internet connection to transmit data, used in the P-Series (Compumedics, Charlotte, NC, USA), or infrared PC communication used in the Biosaca (Swedsleep AB, Gothenburg, Sweden).[124–149] Video may be an option on many of the level II devices, although consideration should be given to practical application of this function.

Level III and IV Devices

Levels III and IV (by CMS definition) devices typically use similar technologies as level II devices but with fewer channels. Because these devices lack EEG channels, their purpose is limited to detecting sleep-disordered breathing. With fewer signals and lack of redundancy, each channel then becomes more important to the final clinical assessment. To optimize ease of use and lightweight design, many devices have software that obtains multiple data signals from a single transducer or lead, although the risk is that the loss of one lead may result in the loss of multiple channels. Variations on snore detectors have been developed. The MediByte products (BRAEBON, Kanata, ON, Canada)[17–19] NOMAD (Nihon Kohden, Tokyo, Japan), and Embletta Gold (Embla, Thornton, CO, USA)[46–55] derive snore signal from the pressure transducer, the SleepScout, SleepView (CleveMed),[20–26] and the ApneaLink devices (ResMed, San Diego, CA, USA)[105–107] derive snore signal from the airflow sensors, whereas others have microphones for the snore channel, which may be located away from the nasal sensors. Conversely, the NovaSom QSG (NovaSom, Glen Burnie, MD, USA)[97–101] derives the airflow signal from noise recorded from microphones overlying the nose and mouth, that is separate from an ambient sound (snore) microphone. The Nox-T3 (CareFusion, San Diego, CA, USA) (Hilmarsson O, Saevarsson G. Validation of automatic analysis in the Noxturnal software for identifying patients with obstructive sleep apnea syndrome (OSAS); Sigurgunnarsdottir MO, Arnardottir ES. Validation study of Nox T3 portable system for identifying patients with suspected obstructive sleep apnea (OSAS), unpublished data, supplied by CareFusion) allows audio playback during review of the study. Respiratory effort channels are necessary to distinguish between obstructive and central respiratory events, and at least one effort channel is required for a level III recorder. Most devices use belt sensors on the thorax or abdomen to detect respiratory effort. The ARES Unicorder (Watermark Medical, Boca Raton, FL, USA)[150–175] detects respiratory effort through a combined signal using pressure transducer sensing forehead venous pressure, venous volume by photoplethysmography, and actigraphy.[61] Computer algorithms may be used in many devices to detect periodic breathing.

Actigraphy and body position are sometimes used to suggest sleep versus wakefulness in devices that do not measure EEG. Most devices that use these channels do so with an accelerometer. However, other technologies have also been developed. The HC1000P software (see later discussion) analyzes changes in the ECG rhythm to determine both body position and sleep state. The WatchPAT (see later discussion) defines sleep state and arousals based on changes in peripheral arterial tone. The Biosaca device (Swedsleep AB) uses a sensor pad placed under the mattress. This pad collects data on ballistic forces on the heart (ballistocardiography), body movement, and respiratory movements, from which sleeper presence, respiratory effort, activity, periodic limb movements, and sleep quality can be determined.

Devices Using Nontraditional Methods

Nontraditional methods of screening for sleep-disordered breathing have become more common as understanding has improved concerning the cardiovascular effects of sleep apnea. ECG-based devices include the Lifescreen Apnea (Spacelabs Healthcare, Issaquah, WA, USA),[120–123] LX Sleep (NorthEast Monitoring, Maynard, MA, USA),[93–96] and HC1000P software (HypnoCore, Yehud, Israel),[56–65] and the M1 Sleep Quality Recorder (Embla).[34–45] Each system uses an algorithm to assess changes in the ECG rhythm and waveforms and associate them with respiratory events, sleep state, or body position. The HC1000P, Lifescreen Apnea, and LX Sleep are software designed for use with ECG Holter monitors with or without oximeters, and use similar analysis methods for detecting OSA from the ECG rhythm. Briefly, the ECG (measured at the skin) is influenced by the respiratory cycle. Movement of the electrodes relative to the heart changes the electrical impedance because of variation in the volume of intrathoracic air. This effect is seen grossly as a slow modulation of the ECG amplitude in sync with the respiratory cycle. The recording is divided into 60-second epochs and, using time-dependant spectral analysis (or power spectral density estimate) of R-R intervals, each epoch is designated either "normal" or "sleep-disordered breathing" (based on the probability that an event has occurred during that epoch).

The LX Sleep and HC1000P combine this ECG analysis with concurrent oximetry data to further categorize sleep-disordered breathing events, allowing categorization as level IV devices. The LX Sleep (in the OxyHolter/A mode) also measures airflow, thereby categorizing it as a level III device. The HC1000P software reportedly can also detect arousals, awakenings, sleep stages (rapid eye movement sleep, light sleep, and slow wave sleep), and respiratory disturbance index through analysis of heart rate variability, body position through analysis of R-wave duration, and electromyography. The M1 Sleep Quality Recorder makes use of a phenomenon known as cardiopulmonary coupling (CPC). During normal non–rapid eye movement sleep, the heart rate is coupled with respiration at a frequency of 0.1 to 0.4 Hz, but the synchronization becomes disrupted and the CPC occurs at lower frequencies (0.01–0.1 Hz) in poor or unstable sleep (as may be seen with OSA, periodic limb movement disorder, or other conditions associated with frequent arousals). REM sleep is associated with very low frequency CPC. In patients with sleep-disordered breathing, narrow-band elevated low frequency

Table 2
Specifications of portable monitoring devices[a]

United States Distributor	Model	Level of PM	Channels	Software	Setup	Maximum Recommended Recording Time	Size	Computer Interface	Power Source	Contact
AGC Biomedical Devices	ApLab	IV[b]	1	ApLab Viewer	Written patient instructions	8 h	81 × 69 × 26 mm 91 g	USB	Internal rechargeable battery	www.agcbiomed.com 800-621-1603
BRAEBON / Fisher & Paykel Healthcare	MediByte[17–19]	III	12	MediByte	Demonstrate in person, video	24 h or 2 nights	71 × 76 × 19 mm 83 g (with battery)	USB	3.6V ½ AA Li battery	www.braebon.com 888-462-4841
	MediByte Jr[17–19]	III	6	MediByte	Demonstrate in person, video	24 h or 2 nights	71 × 76 × 19 mm 81 g (with battery)	USB	3.6V ½ AA Li battery	www.braebon.com 888-462-4841
Cadwell Laboratories	ApneaTrak	III	9	Easy III; Web portal[c]	Written patient instructions, color-coded connector & input, LED feedback to patient	20 h	96 × 89 × 22 mm 122 g	USB	Rechargeable internal NiMH battery	800-245-3001
	Easy Ambulatory PSG	II	32	Easy III	Technician setup	Up to 6 d	191 × 114 × 38 mm 544 g (with battery)	Ethernet	2 × C or D cell battery	www.cadwell.com 800-245-3001
CareFusion	NOX-T3[d]	III	14	NOXturnal	Written and visual patient instructions	>30 h	79 × 63 × 21 mm 88 g (with battery)	USB	1 × AA (alkaline or NiMH rechargeable) battery	www.carefusion.com 800-231-2466
CleveMed	SleepScout[20–26]	III	9	Crystal PSG; eCrystal PSG[c]	Written and DVD patient instructions	23 h	117 × 69 × 25 mm 190 g (with batteries)	Wireless, USB, Secure Digital card	2 × Li AA batteries	www.CleveMed.com 877-253-8363
	SleepView[20–26]	III	7	Crystal PSG; eCrystal PSG[c]	Written and DVD patient instructions, feedback to patient about data quality	Up to 6 nights	76 × 56 × 18 mm 57 g (with batteries)	USB	1 × AAA battery	www.CleveMed.com 877-253-8363
	Sapphire PSG + DreamPort[21–27]	II	22	Crystal PSG; eCrystal PSG[c]	Technician setup, remote monitoring	12 h	213 × 102 × 35 mm 538 g (with batteries)	Wireless/cellular, USB, Secure Digital card	4 × AA batteries	www.CleveMed.com 877-253-8363
	Crystal Monitor PSG Series + DreamPort[21–28]	II	14	Crystal PSG; eCrystal PSG[c]	Technician setup, remote monitoring	12 h	133 × 64 × 26 mm 210 g (with batteries)	Wireless/cellular, USB, Secure Digital card	2 × Li AA batteries	www.CleveMed.com 877-253-8363

Manufacturer	Device			Software	Instructions	Recording time	Dimensions/Weight	Connectivity	Power	Contact
Compumedics	Somté	III	8	Somté; ProFusion PSG	Video instructions	30 h	200 g	Compact Flash card, Bluetooth wireless	2 × AA (alkaline or NiMH rechargeable) batteries	www.compumedics.com 877-717-3975
	Somté PSG	II	27	ProFusion PSG	Video instructions	24 h	113 × 65 × 30 mm and 53 × 133 × 25 mm 205 g (w/o batteries)	Ethernet, Bluetooth wireless	2 × AA (alkaline or NiMH rechargeable) batteries	www.compumedics.com 877-717-3975
	P-Series (PS2 Plus)[29–33]	II	18–26	ProFusion PSG	Technician setup	15 h	—	Serial port, modem, or Internet	9V DC power supply or NiMH rechargeable battery	www.compumedics.com 877-717-3975
Embla	M1 Sleep Quality Recorder[34–45]	IV	4	SleepImage[c]	Automatic start with ECG signal	6 × 8-h recordings	79 × 48 × 13 mm 23 g	USB	2 × CR2016 coin cell batteries	www.sleepimage.com
	Embletta Gold[46–55]	III	14	RemLogic-E	Patient hook-up card and DVD	24 h	23 × 71 × 140 mm 218 g	USB, serial port	Built-in rechargeable batteries	www.embla.com 888-662-7632
	Embla titanium[46–55]	I	34	RemLogic[g]; Somnologica	Technician setup	>24 h	89 × 191 × 290 mm 200 g	Ethernet/USB, wireless, Compact Flash card	2 × AA batteries	www.embla.com 888-662-7632
	Embletta X100[46–55]	II	14	Somnologica Studio	Technician setup	24 h	20 × 65 × 124 mm and 15 × 20 × 53 mm 146 g with batteries and 60 g	USB, serial port	2 × AA alkaline or rechargeable batteries	www.embla.com 888-662-7632
Grass Technologies	AURA PSG	II	25	TWin[g]	Technician setup, programmable start time	10 h (wireless), 12 h (ambulatory)	89 × 158 × 25 mm 280 g	Compact Flash card, Ethernet, Bluetooth wireless	3.6V Li rechargeable battery	www.grasstechnologies.com 877-472-7779
	AURA PSG LITE	II	16	TWin[g]	Technician setup, programmable start time	10 h (wireless), 12 h (ambulatory)	89 × 158 × 25 mm 280 g	Compact Flash card, Ethernet, Bluetooth wireless	3.6V Li rechargeable battery	www.grasstechnologies.com 877-472-7779
	SleepTrek 3	III	6	GammaST; TWin[g]	Written and video patient instructions	12+ h	89 × 158 × 25 mm 280 g	Compact Flash card	3.6V Li rechargeable battery	www.grasstechnologies.com 877-472-7779

(continued on next page)

Table 2

(continued)

United States Distributor	Model	Level of PM	Channels	Software	Setup	Maximum Recommended Recording Time	Size	Computer Interface	Power Source	Contact
HypnoCore	Any available continuous ECG and pulse-ox device	IV	2	HC1000P[56-65]	e	e	e	e	e	www.hypnocore.com +972-73-2903400
Individual Monitoring Systems	SleepCheck[f,66-70]	IV[b]	1	None (direct readout)	Machine feedback to patient	9 h	76 × 51 × 9 mm 55 g (with battery)	N/A	1 × AAA battery	www.imsystems.net 888-513-5969
Itamar Medical	Watch PAT[16,71-87]	IV	6 (peripheral arterial tone)	WatchPAT	Video patient instructions	10 h continuous use	79 × 48 × 20 mm 130 g	USB	Rechargeable Li ion battery	www.itamar-medical.com 888-748-2627
Jant Pharmacal	Accutest SleepStrip[88-92]	N/A	1	None (direct readout)	Instruction manual; feedback to patient if time too short	8.5 h	160 × 35 × 3.5 mm 9 g	N/A	Miniature 3V Li battery	www.accutest.net 800-676-5565
LifeWatch Services	Nitewatch	III	6	NiteWatch Connect[c]	Representative calls the patient	3 d	85 g	Cellular	—	www.nitewatchservices.com 877-246-6483
Natus Medical	Trex Home Sleep	II	34	SleepWorks	Technician setup	96 h	155 × 102 × 25 mm 312 g	USB	2 × AA batteries	www.natus.com 800-303-0306
Nihon Kohden America	Nomad	III	11	Polysmith	Automatic start with valid pulse signal, color-coded sensors	17 h	117 × 72 × 25 mm 180 g (without batteries)	USB, Bluetooth	2 × AA batteries	www.nkusa.com 800-325-0283
	Trackit (18/8 or 24P) ± Sleep-Click-on	II	28-32	Insight II and Reveal; NK1200, NK9200; Polysmith[g]	Technician setup, auto-start with valid pulse signal	96 h	140 × 95 × 3 mm <500 g (with batteries)	USB, serial port	3 × 9V Li batteries or one high capacity rechargeable battery	www.llines.com www.lifelinesneuro.com 800-325-0283
	Trackit Sleep Walker	II	16	Trackit; Polysmith[g]	Technician setup, auto-start with valid pulse signal	30 h	140 × 90 × 35 mm <400 g (with batteries)	USB, Bluetooth	1-3 × 9V batteries	www.llines.com 800-325-0283

Manufacturer	Device	Level	No.	Software	Patient instructions	Recording time	Dimensions/weight	Data transfer	Power	Contact
NorthEast Monitoring	DR180 Series / OxyHolter	III	4	LX Sleep, compatible with Holter LX Analysis[91–94]	Technician setup	72 h with Li batteries 48 h with alkaline 24 h with rechargeable	120 × 70 × 25 mm 200 g (with batteries)	Compact Flash card (DR180+), Secure Digital card (DR181)	2 × AA batteries (alkaline, rechargeable, or Li)	www.nemon.com 866-346-5837
NovaSom	NovaSom QSG[97–101]	III	3	NovaSom Study Viewer	Voice prompts, video, written instructions	>3 × 8-h nights	217 × 185 × 71 mm + 100 × 72 × 29 mm 964 + 116 g	N/A (shipped by patient, report on secure Web site)	AC power	www.novasom.com 877-753-3775
Philips Respironics	RUSleeping RTS Screener[f,66–70]	IV[b]	1	None (direct readout)	Written patient instructions	9 h	76 × 51 × 9 mm 48 g (without battery)	N/A	1 × AAA alkaline battery	www.philips.com/respironics 800-345-6443
	Alice PDx[102]	II–III	21	Sleepware	Color-coded diagram and labels, patient feedback	18–20 h	127 × 76 × 51 mm 230 g (without batteries)	USB	3 × AA alkaline batteries	www.philips.com/respironics 800-345-6443
	Stardust II[103,104]	III	7	Stardust Host	Written patient instructions	8.5 h	115 × 58 × 20 mm 102 g	Serial port	1 × 9V alkaline battery	www.philips.com/respironics 800-345-6443
ResMed	ApneaLink[105–107]	IV	3	ApneaLink	Video patient instructions	8 h minimum	125 × 60 × 30 mm 50 g (without batteries)	USB	2 × AA (alkaline or NiMH rechargeable) batteries	www.resmed.com 800-424-0737
	ApneaLink Plus[105–107]	III	4	ApneaLink	Video patient instructions	8 h minimum	125 × 60 × 30 mm 50 g (without batteries)	USB	2 × AA (alkaline or NiMH rechargeable) batteries	www.resmed.com 800-424-0737
SagaTech	Remmers Sleep Recorder[108]	III	8	Online Sleep Portal[c]	Machine feedback to patient	3 nights	50 × 190 × 205 mm 1000 g	Serial port or USB	AC power	www.sagatech.ca 403-228-4214
SNAP Diagnostics	SNAP Test[4,109]	III	7	SNAP; SNAP Web portal[c]	Written and video patient instructions	No recommended maximum	35 × 140 × 102 mm 451 g	USB	AC power, built-in rechargeable battery	www.snapdiagnostics.com 800-762-7786

(continued on next page)

Table 2
(continued)

United States Distributor	Model	Level of PM	Channels	Software	Setup	Maximum Recommended Recording Time	Size	Computer Interface	Power Source	Contact
SOMNOmedics	SOMNOwatch plus (EEG 6 or RESP)[h,110–112]	II	13	DOMINO[g]	Programmable start and end times	46–80 h	45 mm diameter × 16 mm 30 g (with battery) and 61 × 56 × 13 mm, 60 g for EEG 6	USB	Rechargeable Li ion battery	www.somnomedics-diagnostics.com 866-361-9937
	SOMNOscreen Plus[112–119]	II	33	DOMINO[g]	Technician setup, delayed automatic start	36 h	140 × 70 × 28 mm 220 g (with battery)	Compact Flash card, wireless	Rechargeable Li ion battery	www.somnomedics-diagnostics.com 866-361-9937
	SOMNOscreen EEG 10–20 PSG[112–119]	II	43	DOMINO[g]	Technician setup, programmable start and end times	24 h	140 × 70 × 28 mm 260 g (with battery)	Online (wireless or cable), Compact Flash card	Rechargeable Li ion battery	www.somnomedics-diagnostics.com 866-361-9937
Spacelabs Health care	Lifecard CF	IV[b]	1	Lifescreen Apnea[120–123]	Technician setup	7 d	96 × 57 × 18 mm 118 g	Compact Flash card	1 × AAA alkaline or rechargeable NiMH battery	www.spacelabshealthcare.com 425-657-7200
Swedsleep AB	Biosaca[124–149]	II	22	Sleep Studio; Monit[g]	Technician setup	19–25 h	206 × 115 × 49 mm and 77 × 62 × 13 mm 650 g (with batteries)	Infrared, Compact Flash card	6 × AA batteries	www.swedsleep.se +46 (0)31-10 77 80
Watermark Medical	ARES Uni-corder[150–175]	III	7	Watermark Medical Sleep Study Portal[e]	Video and written patient instructions	21 h	64 × 51 × 25 mm 113 g (with battery)	USB	2 250 mAh 3.7V Li ion rechargeable batteries	www.watermarkmedical.com 877-710-6999

Abbreviations: LED, light emitting diode; Li, lithium; N/A, not applicable; NiMH, nickel-metal hydride; PM, portable monitoring; PSG, polysomnography.

[a] Detailed information presented here is largely based on the manufacturers' and distributors' literature.

[b] Meets AASM, but not CMS, definition of type IV device (ie, do not allow for calculation of RDI or AHI using at least three channels).

[c] Remote storage, scoring, and/or interpretation via Internet.

[d] Omar Hilmarsson, Gudmundur Saevarsson. Validation of automatic analysis in the Noxturnal software for identifying patients with obstructive sleep apnea syndrome (OSAS): Magdalena Osk Sigurgunnarsdottir, Erna Sif Arnardottir. Validation study of Nox T3 portable system for identifying patients with suspected obstructive sleep apnea (OSAS), unpublished data, supplied by CareFusion.

[e] HypnoCore HC1000P makes use of available pulse oximeter and ECG devices, therefore setup and device specifications vary based on the type of device used.

[f] SleepCheck and RUSleeping RTS are equivalent devices manufactured and distributed under agreements by Individual Monitoring Systems and Philips Respironics, respectively.

[g] Data can be stored in European Data Format (EDF) and may be compatible with other interpretation software programs.

[h] Device is not yet approved by the US Food and Drug Administration.

coupling (ie, clustering of the low frequency CPC events at or near a few frequencies) is seen with periodic central or obstructive patterns, and may be obscured by more overt OSA, but is uncovered once positive airway pressure is initiated. The snore detector and body position monitor may help in diagnosing sleep-disordered breathing.

The WatchPAT (Itamar Medical, Caesarea, Israel)[16,71] makes use of the vascular changes associated with sleep and sleep apnea, measured with peripheral arterial tonometry. This method measures arterial pulse wave volume in the finger. Reduction in pulse amplitude indicates peripheral vasoconstriction and is a surrogate measure of sympathetic activation. It is used in combination with an accelerometer to determine wake/sleep and a pulse oximeter. An attenuation of the pulse amplitude, combined with acceleration of the pulse rate or increase in wrist activity, signifies an arousal or respiratory event. A respiratory event is also scored if pulse amplitude reduction occurs in combination with oxygen desaturation.

Advantages to the nontraditional methods include patient comfort (no sensors near the head or face) and cardiovascular monitoring during the study. Disadvantages of these devices lie in their indirect methods of measuring respiratory patterns. None of these devices measure airflow, respiratory effort, or sleep state (using EEG) but rather rely on physiologic changes related to those events. The results, although potentially sensitive and specific for detecting sleep-disordered breathing, are not equivalent to those derived from more traditional methods. Additionally, they generally cannot be used in patients with chronic arrhythmias, such as atrial fibrillation, heart block, or ventricular pacing.

EVALUATION OF PM DEVICES

The type of PM chosen for use in a medical practice to diagnose an individual patient should be based on current and anticipated needs and resources available. Although no formal criteria exist for evaluating PM devices, the authors suggest using criteria outlined in **Box 1**. Important factors relating to the patient, clinician, or the device itself may make a specific device more attractive in a given circumstance.

Patient-relevant factors are more directly related to what concerns the patient; however, they are also important to the clinician. If the instructions are simple to follow or the device has cues that provide feedback, patients will be more likely to use a device properly and obtain adequate data, especially with devices patients set up themselves. By contrast, patients may be less likely to sleep with

an uncomfortable, intrusive device, thereby making the study less adequate. If a case such as this involves a level III or IV recorder that does not allow for sleep detection, the recording time will be the same, but the severity of sleep-disordered breathing will be more substantially underestimated because the time asleep will constitute a smaller proportion of the total recording time. With level II devices, the sleep time recorded will be shorter, possibly compromising the quality of the study. Devices that can be set up by the patient in the home require fewer staff resources from the sleep laboratory. However, at least one staff member must be well trained in the use of the device. Patients may need to be instructed on the use of the device, the devices need to be cleaned and maintained, and problems that arise during the studies may need troubleshooting.

For many of the more complex home sleep test devices, especially those that require application of EEG or ECG leads, patients must come into the office or sleep center for a staff member to perform the setup. Alternatively, the staff member can go to the patient's home to set up the study; this reduces the likelihood of incorrect setup and allows for verification of proper functioning, such as checking impedances. This method also requires additional staffing and is often performed during the day, meaning the patient must wear the device until bedtime, which can be uncomfortable and increases the chances that one or more leads will detach. Devices that are mailed or delivered to the patient are more convenient for the patient but may reduce the level of control over study quality. Most PM devices require patients to either return the device through the mail or deliver it to the clinic. Alternatively, a staff member may need to go back to the patient's home to collect the machine. The easier the return process is for patients, the more likely the device will be returned in a timely manner.

Lastly, it is important for patients to know what to do when things go wrong during the study. If a sensor comes off during the night, or the patient takes it off, instructions on how to replace it should be provided; this can be done with the instruction manual. If a more difficult problem arises during the night, a reliable contact should be available, such as a night technologist working at the sleep laboratory or personnel from one of the PM companies offering 24-hour support.

Clinician-relevant factors are equally important in determining the appropriate device to use, and these affect care delivered to the patient. It is important for clinicians to choose a device with the appropriate number and type of channels for the intended purposes. A level IV device lacking respiratory effort channels would probably not be

Table 3
Components of individual home sleep testing devices[a]

	Level	EEG	No. EEG Channels	EOG	Chin EMG	ECG	Airflow Sensor (Type)	Respiratory Effort Sensor (Type)	Oxygen Saturation/ Pulse Rate	Limb EMG	Body Position	Actigraphy	Miscellaneous	United States Distributor
ApLab	IV[b]						+ (NP)							AGC Biomedical Devices
MediByte	III					+	+ (NP and therm)	+ (Thor and abd)	+	+			Audio	BRAEBON / Fisher & Paykel Healthcare
MediByte Jr	III				+		+ (NP)	+ (Thor)	+		+			
ApneaTrak	III						+ (NP and therm)	+ (Thor and abd)	+	+	+		Snore from NP and sound	Cadwell Laboratories
Easy Ambulatory PSG	II	+	11	+	+	+	+ (NP and therm)	+ (Thor and abd)	+		+	+	Snore audio	
NOX-T3	III	c	c	c	c	c	+ (NP)	+ (Thor and abd)	+		+	+	Snore audio, two optional ExG channels; wireless pulse-oximetry	CareFusion
SleepScout	III	+		+	+	+	+ (NP)	+ (Thor and abd)	+		+		Snore from NP	CleveMed
SleepView	III						+ (NP and therm)	+ (Thor)	+		+			
Sapphire PSG (wireless)	II	+	6	+	+	+	+ (NP and therm)	+ (Thor and abd)	+	+	+		etCO2 channel, Dreamport for portable	
Crystal Monitor PSG Series	II	+	4	+	+	+	+ (NP and therm)	+ (Thor and abd)	+	+	+		Dreamport for portable	
Somté	III	c		c	c	+	+ (NP)	+ (Thor and abd)	+	+	+		Two ExG channels	Compumedics
Somté PSG	II	+	2	+	+	+	+ (NP and therm)	+ (Thor and abd)	+	+	+	+		
P-Series (PS2 plus)	II	+		+	+	+	+ (NP and therm)	+ (Thor and abd)	+	+	+		Light sensor, tracheal microphone	
M1 Sleep Quality Recorder	IV					+	+ (derive from ECG)	+ (derive from ECG)				+		Embla
Embletta	II	+		+	+	+	+ (NP and therm)	+ (Thor and abd)			+	+		

Device	Type	EEG	No. of channels	EOG	EMG	ECG	Airflow	Respiratory effort	Oximetry	Body position	Comments	Manufacturer
Embla titanium	II	+	12	+	+	+	+ (NP and therm)	+ (Thor and abd)	+	+		
Embletta X100	II	+	2	+	+	+	+ (NP)	+ (Thor and abd)	+	+		
AURA PSG	II	+	8	+	+	+	+ (NP and therm)	+ (Thor and abd)	+		Snore; pulse transit time; CO_2 and pH available	Grass Technologies
SleepTrek 3	III			+		+	+ (NP)	+ (Thor)	+		Snore; patient-worn multi-sensor	
AURA PSG LITE	II	+	4	+		+	+ (NP and therm)	+ (Thor and abd)	+		Snore; pulse transit time	
SleepCheck	IV[b]					+	+ (NP)		+		No data download	IM systems
WatchPAT 200	IV					+			+	+	PAT, snore	Itamar Medical
Accutest SleepStrip	IV[b]						+ (Therm)				No data download	Jant Pharmacal
NiteWatch	III			+		+	+	+	+		Snore	LifeWatch Services
Trex	II	+	24	+	+	+	+ (NP and therm)	+	+		Ambulatory video	Natus Medical
Trackit 18/8 (24P) + Sleep Click-On	II	+	18 + 8 (20 + 4)	+	+	+	+	+ (Thor and abd)	+		Video link	Nihon Kohden America
Trackit Sleep Walker	II	+	4	+	+	+	+ (NP)	+ (Thor and abd)	+			
Nomad	III			+	+	+	+ (NP and therm)	+ (Thor and abd)	+			
LX Sleep (DR180 Series, OxyHolter, or/ OxyHolter/A)	III					+	+ (OxyHolter/A: therm)	+ (ECG-derived respiratory signal)	+			NorthEast Monitoring
NovaSom	III						+ (NP)	+ (Thor)	+			NovaSom
RUSleeping RTS Screener	IV[b]	c		c			+ (NP)		+			Phillips Respironics
Alice PDx	II–III	c		c		+	+ (NP and therm)	+ (Thor and abd)	+		Optional ExG; real-time view	
Stardust II	III					+	+ (NP)	+ (Thor)	+		Real-time view	
ApneaLink	IV					+	+ (NP)		+			ResMed

(continued on next page)

Table 3
(continued)

	Level	EEG	No. EEG Channels	EOG	Chin EMG	ECG	Airflow Sensor (Type)	Respiratory Effort Sensor (Type)	Oxygen Saturation/ Pulse Rate	Limb EMG	Body Position	Actigraphy	Miscellaneous	United States Distributor
ApneaLink Plus	III						+ (NP)	+ (Thor)	+					
Remmers Sleep Recorder	III						+ (NP)	+	+	+	+		Snore count	Sagatech
SNAP Test	III						+	+	+		+		sound	Snap diagnostics
SOMNOscreen plus	II	+	10	+	+	+	+ (NP and therm)	+ (Thor and abd)	+	+	+		Ambient light sensor	SOMNOmedics
SOMNOwatch plus (EEG 6 or RESP)	II–III	+ (EEG 6 only)	6	+ (EEG 6 only)	+ (EEG 6 only)	+ (EEG 6 only)	+ (NP)	+ (Thor and abd)	+		+		Ambient light sensor, waterproof	
SOMNOscreen II EEG 10–20	II	+	25	+	+	+	+ (NP and therm)	+ (Thor)	+	+	+		Ambient light sensor	
Biosaca	II	+	16	+	+	+	+ (Therm)	+ (User-defined)	+	+	+		Sound, BCG Sensor Pad; video	Swedsleep AB
Lifescreen Apnea	IV[b]					+	+ (derive from ECG)	+ (derive from ECG)						Spacelabs Helathcare
ARES	III	+[c]	[c]				+ (NP)	+ (Thor)	+				Head position, optional two EEG channels	Watermark Medical

Abbreviations: Abd, abdominal effort channel; BCG, Ballisto CardioGraphy; etCO$_2$, end-tidal carbon dioxide channel; ExG, generic channels for EEG, ECG, or EOG; ECG, electrocardiography; EEG, electroencephalography; EOG, electrooculography; NP, nasal pressure channel; PAT, peripheral arterial tonometry; Therm, thermistor airflow channel; Thor, thoracic effort channel.

[a] Information based on manufacturers' Web sites and product brochures.

[b] Do not meet Centers for Medicare & Mediaid criteria for level IV (fewer than three channels).

[c] Optional EEG/ExG channels available.

Box 1
Portable monitoring device evaluation factors

1. Patient-relevant factors

   a. Ease of operation

      i. Bedtime application
      ii. Disconnect/reconnect during the night

   b. Ease of assembly (if needed at home) or requires technician setup
   c. Clarity and user-friendliness of operator manual
   d. Portability of device (mail, return to clinic, in-home pick-up)
   e. Intrusiveness (noise, light, discomfort)
   f. Support (24-hour service)

2. Clinician-relevant factors

   a. Ease and completeness of scoring software

      i. Appropriate leads (category of device)
      ii. Compatibility with operating systems
      iii. Range of events detected
      iv. Quality of automatic scoring
      v. Need for additional software that is compatible with existing polysomnography software, or a Web portal
      vi. Computer interface (card, USB, wireless/Internet)

   b. Ease of cleaning for reuse
   c. Ease of instruction to patient (clinic, in-home demonstration)
   d. Accessibility of tech support and quality of service

3. Device-specific factors

   a. Length of warranty
   b. Quality of the parts

      i. Leads
      ii. Contacts

   c. Cost of device and software

      i. Initial costs
      ii. Replacement parts versus reusable
      iii. Software updates
      iv. Reimbursement

appropriate to use in a population with a high prevalence of periodic breathing. By contrast, a level II device with EEG may be overkill in an obese, snoring, hypertensive man who regularly falls asleep notwithstanding 8 hours of bedtime nightly. Determining the patient population's needs before investing in a PM device is worthwhile.

The ability to "turn over" a device between patients becomes important in high-volume clinics. Therefore, the ease of cleaning, replacing parts,

and changing or charging the batteries becomes key. Alkaline batteries are quick to replace but add to the cost of using the device, whereas rechargeable batteries require more time (to recharge). When considering investing in a device, the reliability of a company's technical support and the quality of the service, if known, should be taken into account when one is embarking on a potentially long-term relationship with the company.

The quality of the review software affects the ease and accuracy of diagnosis. Most PM devices ship with automatic scoring software; however, current guidelines require that the raw data are available for review. Studies comparing PM devices with standard PSG have used the automatic scoring for analysis. In most cases, the computerized results reasonably approximate manual scoring by experienced technologists. Sleep medicine specialists are more likely to review raw data; therefore, software presenting the data in a familiar layout (ie, similar to PSG) may be preferred. In some cases, a PM device may use software that a clinician has already acquired for use with laboratory PSG studies, thereby simplifying the process of reviewing the data and generating reports. Level II devices typically can be used for full PSG, and therefore use identical display and analysis software. Level III and IV devices that share PSG software include the SleepScout and SleepView (CleveMed), Somté (Compumedics), SleepTrek 3 (Grass Technologies, West Warwick, RI, USA), and Trex Home Sleep (Natus, San Carlos, CA, USA). The Trackit devices (Nihon Kohden) and Biosaca (Swedsleep AB) record data in native European Data Format (EDF) or can convert data to EDF, allowing transport to software review systems. Clinicians interested mainly in the final outcome may prefer simple, easy-to-use automatic scoring systems or online Web portals that have the ability to analyze data and generate reports.

An additional option would be the use of a full-service PM company that handles everything, including mailing the device to the patient, analyzing the data, and generating the report. Some of these companies are also accredited as sleep laboratories, allowing them to manage the diagnostic process once the referral is placed. If using a Web portal to upload data, patient confidentiality remains vital. All connections must be secure and the site receiving the information should provide assurances of security and confidentiality. The type of computer interface for uploading the data is important. Some are faster than others, which can affect processing efficiency, especially for large studies. Although most software is compatible with PC-based Windows, a few are available for use on Mac or other platforms. This availability changes constantly, and therefore contacting the vendor for current status is important.

Device-specific factors should not be marginalized. These factors can radically change the experience of using a device. No device is intended to break down, but what warranty coverage is available is important to know. The cost of the replaceable parts varies among devices and can reduce net income for studies. Higher-quality parts would be expected to require less frequent replacements; however, no easily accessible method exists though which quality and durability of devices can be compared. Reusable parts should be expected to last longer and cost more than disposable parts. Updates to the review software can add unexpected costs, unless they are provided free by the distributor or covered by the original purchase agreement. Lastly, reimbursement for tests performed with the device will vary according to the type of device. If home sleep testing is intended to generate profit, it is important to research not only current reimbursement rates versus costs but also the prior and predicted trends.

SUMMARY

The choice of PM device to use for nonlaboratory diagnosis of OSA depends on many factors. Each device is unique in the spectrum of data acquired and quality of the analyzing software. In addition to clinical factors, the ease of use and the support provided by the company can make an enormous difference in using these devices for patient care. Numerous clinical studies have compared PM devices with PSG. No significant studies have yet compared PM devices in terms of clinical impact. Therefore, the choice among devices should be made based on need and available resources. Tabular information in this article is based on literature provided directly by device distributors and data published in journal articles.

REFERENCES

1. Young T, Peppard PE, Gottlieb DJ. Epidemiology of obstructive sleep apnea: a population health perspective. Am J Respir Crit Care Med 2002; 165:1217–39.

2. Young T, Palta M, Dempsey J, et al. The occurrence of sleep-disordered breathing among middle-aged adults. N Engl J Med 1993;328:1230–5.

3. American Academy of Sleep Medicine. Sleep-related breathing disorders in adults: recommendations for syndrome definition and measurement techniques in clinical research; the report of an American Academy of Sleep Medicine task force. Sleep 1999;22:667–89.

4. Su S, Baroody FM, Kohrman M, et al. A comparison of polysomnography and a portable home sleep study in the diagnosis of obstructive sleep apnea syndrome. Otolaryngol Head Neck Surg 2004; 131:844–50.

5. Ferber R, Millman R, Coppola M, et al. Portable recording in the assessment of obstructive sleep apnea: ASDA standards of practice. Sleep 1994; 17:378–92.

6. American Sleep Disorders Association. Practice parameters for the indications for polysomnography and related procedures: polysomnography Task Force, American Sleep Disorders Association Standards of Practice Committee. Sleep 1997;20: 406–22.

7. Chesson AL, Ferber RA, Fry JM, et al. The indications for polysomnography and related procedures. Sleep 1997;20:423–87.

8. Collop N, Anderson W, Boehlecke B, et al. Clinical guidelines for the use of unattended portable monitors in the diagnosis of obstructive sleep apnea in adult patients. J Clin Sleep Med 2007;3:737–47.

9. Agency for Healthcare Research and Quality. Technology assessment: home diagnosis of Obstructive Sleep Apnea-Hypopnea Syndrome. Available at: http://www.cms.hhs.gov/determinationprocess/downloads/id48TA.pdf. Accessed June 22, 2011.

10. Orr WC, Eiken T, Pegram V, et al. A laboratory validation study of a portable system for remote recording of sleep-related breathing disorders. Chest 1994;105:160–2.

11. Emsellem HA, Corson WA, Rappaport BA, et al. Verification of sleep apnea using a portable sleep apnea screening device. South Med J 1990;83:748–52.

12. Ancoli-Israel S, Kripke DF, Mason W, et al. Comparisons of home sleep recordings and polysomnograms in older adults with sleep disorders. Sleep 1981;4:283–91.

13. Gyulay S, Gould D, Sawyer B, et al. Evaluation of a microprocessor-based portable home monitoring system to measure breathing during sleep. Sleep 1987;10:130–42.

14. Trikalinos TA, Ip S, Raman G, et al. Home diagnosis of obstructive sleep apnea-hypopnea syndrome. Department of Health & Human Services. Agency for Healthcare Research and Quality; 2007. Available at: http://www.ahrq.gov/clinic/techix.htm#competed. Accessed June 22, 2011.

15. Morgenthaler T, Alessi C, Friedman L, et al. Practice parameters for the use of actigraphy in the assessment of sleep and sleep disorders: an update for 2007. Sleep 2007;30(4):519–29.

16. Pittman SD, Ayas NT, MacDonald MM, et al. Using a wrist-worn device based on peripheral arterial tonometry to diagnose obstructive sleep

apnea: in-laboratory and ambulatory validation. Sleep 2004;27(5):923–33.

17. Driver HS, Pereira EJ, Bjerring K, et al. Validation of the MediByte Type 3 portable monitor compared with polysomnography for screening of obstructive sleep apnea. Can Respir J 2011;18(3):137–43.

18. Helen DS, Bjerring KA, Stewart SC, et al. Pilot evaluation of a portable monitor for diagnosis of obstructive sleep apnea in a consecutive series of patients compared with polysomnography [abstract]. Sleep 2008;31(Suppl):1035.

19. Carlile JB. Comparison between level III portable monitoring system and PSG on 44 in lab patients [abstract]. Sleep 2010;33(Abstract Suppl):0413.

20. Kayyali H, Bellezza T, Weimer S, et al. Self-administered wireless monitor for comprehensive evaluation of CPAP benefit in the home. Sleep Diag Ther 2010;5(2):44–9.

21. Weimer S, Kayyali H, Frederick C, et al. Innovative wireless sleep disorders diagnosis system [abstract]. Sleep 2006;29(Suppl):1026.

22. Kayyali H. Wireless transmission of polysomnography. Presented at Cleveland Clinic: Lung Summit 2006. Cleveland, April 20–22, 2006.

23. Schmidt RN. A new wireless sleep disorders diagnostic device. Presented at Bilingual Pan American Health Care Engineering Conference. Long Beach/Los Angeles, January 30–February 2, 2006.

24. Johnson MW, Guiffrida J, Modarreszadeh M, et al. A novel neonatal telemetry system for sleep monitoring [abstract]. Sleep 2004;27(Suppl):815.

25. Weimer S, Kayyali H, Frederick C, et al. Innovative wireless sleep apnea monitoring system [abstract]. Sleep 2004;27(Suppl):817.

26. Pao J, Tarler M, Frederick C, et al. Neural net based arrhythmia analysis software [abstract]. Sleep 2004;27(Suppl):821.

27. Weimer S, Halley D, Grogan A, et al. Evaluating the radio frequency environment is needed before selecting a wireless PSG system [abstract]. Sleep 2007;30(Suppl):1020.

28. Kayyali HA, Weimer S, Frederick C, et al. Remotely attended home monitoring of sleep disorders. Telemed J E Health 2008;14(4):371–4.

29. Quan SF, Howard BV, Iber C, et al. The Sleep Heart Health Study: design, rationale, and methods. Sleep 1997;20(12):1077–85.

30. Redline S, Sanders MH, Lind BK, et al. Methods for obtaining and analyzing unattended polysomnography data for a multicenter study. Sleep 1998; 21(7):759–67.

31. Whitney CW, Gottlieb DJ, Redline S, et al. Reliability of scoring respiratory disturbance indices and sleep staging. Sleep 1998;21(7):749–57.

32. Kapur VK, Rapoport DM, Sanders MH, et al. Rates of sensor loss in unattended home polysomnography: the influence of age, gender, obesity, and sleep-disordered breathing. Sleep 2000;23(5): 682–8.

33. Nieto FJ, Young TB, Lind BK, et al. Association of sleep-disordered breathing, sleep apnea, and hypertension in a large community-based study. Sleep Heart Health Study. JAMA 2000;283(14): 1829–36.

34. Thomas RJ, Mietus JE, Peng CK, et al. An electrocardiogram-based technique to assess cardiopulmonary coupling during sleep. Sleep 2005;28(9):1151–61.

35. Thomas RJ, Mietus JE, Peng CK, et al. Differentiating obstructive from central and complex sleep apnea using an automated electrocardiogram-based method. Sleep 2007;30(12):1756–69.

36. Thomas RJ, Weiss MD, Mietus JE, et al. Prevalent hypertension and stroke in heart health study: association with an ECG-derived spectrographic marker of cardiopulmonary coupling. Sleep 2009; 32(7):897–904.

37. Schramm P, Baker DN. An electrocardiogram-based technique to identify complex sleep apnea in patients with diabetes and sleep disordered breathing [abstract]. Sleep 2009;33(Suppl):0418.

38. Schramm P, Baker DN, Neville AG, et al. An electrocardiogram-based technique to assess cardiopulmonary coupling during sleep in pediatric patients suspected with sleep disordered breathing [abstract]. Sleep 2009;32(Suppl):0244.

39. Schramm P, Neville AG, Madison S, et al. Cardiopulmonary coupling (CPC) measures correlate to standard sleep variables in a random sample of patients suspected with sleep disordered breathing [abstract]. Sleep 2009;32(Suppl):0575.

40. Schramm P, Baker DN, Neville AN, et al. Cardiopulmonary coupling, a novel method to assess sleep quality: validation in patients suspected with sleep disordered breathing [abstract]. Sleep 2009; 32(Suppl):1142.

41. Thomas RJ, Mietus JE, Peng CK, et al. Impaired sleep quality in fibromyalgia: detection and quantification with ECG-based cardiopulmonary coupling spectrograms. Sleep Med 2010;11(5):497–8.

42. Schramm P. An early indicator of complex sleep apnea. ADVANCE for Respiratory Care & Sleep Medicine. Available at: http://respiratory-care-sleep-medicine.advanceweb.com/Article/An-Early-Indicator-of-Complex-Sleep-Apnea.aspx. Accessed March 14, 2011.

43. Schramm PJ, Neville A, Baker D. The sleep quality recovery of a snorer's bed partner. Respir Ther 2010;5(3):39–40.

44. Yang AC, Yang CH, Hong CJ, et al. Sleep state instabilities in major depressive disorders: detection and quantification with electrocardiogram-based cardiopulmonary coupling analysis. Psychophysiology 2011;48(2):285–91.

45. Ibrahim LH, Jacono FJ, Patel SR, et al. Heritability of abnormalities in cardiopulmonary coupling in sleep apnea: use of an electrocardiogram-based technique. Sleep 2010;33(5):643–6.

46. Zvartau NE, Conrady AO, Sviryaev YV, et al. Marinobufagenin in hypertensive patients with obstructive sleep apnea. Cell Mol Biol 2006;52(8):24–7.

47. Bridevaux PO, Fitting JW, Fellrath JM, et al. Interobserver agreement on apnea hypopnea index using portable monitoring of respiratory parameters. Swiss Med Wkly 2007;137(43–44):602–7.

48. Abdelghani A, Roisman G, Escourrou P. Evaluation of a home respiratory polygraphy system in the diagnosis of the obstructive sleep apnea syndrome. Rev Mal Respir 2007;24(3 Pt 1):331–8 [in French].

49. Oldenburg O, Lamp B, Faber L, et al. Sleep-disordered breathing in patients with symptomatic heart failure: a contemporary study of prevalence in and characteristics of 700 patients. Eur J Heart Fail 2007;9(3):251–7.

50. Shen QB, Xu DL, Lin S, et al. Sleep-disordered breathing and left ventricular remodeling in patients with chronic heart failure. Nan Fang Yi Ke Da Xue Bao 2006;26(4):486–9 [in Chinese].

51. Endeshaw YW, Katz S, Ouslander JG, et al. Association of denture use with sleep-disordered breathing among older adults. J Public Health Dent 2004;64(3):181–3.

52. Decker MJ. Validation of Embla respiration analysis (formerly Medcare) [abstract]. Presented at the American Thoracic Society 100th International Conference. Orlando, May 21–26, 2004.

53. Droitcour AD, Seto TB, Park BK, et al. Non-contact respiratory rate measurement validation for hospitalized patients. Conf Proc IEEE Eng Med Biol Soc 2009;2009:4812–5.

54. Meltzer EO, Munafo DA, Chung W, et al. Intranasal mometasone furoate therapy for allergic rhinitis symptoms and rhinitis-disturbed sleep. Ann Allergy Asthma Immunol 2010;105(1):65–74.

55. Skomro RP, Gjevre J, Reid J, et al. Outcomes of home-based diagnosis and treatment of obstructive sleep apnea. Chest 2010;138(2):257–63.

56. Baharav A, Kotagal S, Gibbons V, et al. Fluctuations in autonomic nervous activity during sleep displayed by power spectrum analysis of heart rate variability. Neurology 1995;45(6):1183–7.

57. Baharav A, Kotagal S, Rubin BK, et al. Autonomic cardiovascular control in children with obstructive sleep apnea. Clin Auton Res 1999;9(6):345–51.

58. Shinar Z, Baharav A, Akselrod S. R wave duration as a measure of body position changes during sleep. Comput Cardiol 1999;26:49–52.

59. Baharav A, Shinar Z, Dagan Y, et al. Impaired autonomic balance during sleep in obstructive sleep apnea: origin or result. Comput Cardiol 2001;28:225–8.

60. Shinar Z, Baharav A, Akselrod S. Changes in autonomic nervous system activity and in electrocortical activity during sleep onset. Comput Cardiol 2003;30:303–6.

61. Shinar Z, Baharav A, Akselrod S. Detection of different recumbent body positions from the electrocardiogram. Med Biol Eng Comput 2003;41(2):206–10.

62. Baharav A, Shinar Z, Sivan Y, et al. Electrocardiogram based evaluation of children with sleep related upper airway obstruction. Comput Cardiol 2004;31:289–92.

63. Furman GD, Shinar Z, Baharav A, et al. Electrocardiogram derived respiration during sleep. Comput Cardiol 2005;32:351–4.

64. Shinar Z, Akselrod S, Dagan Y, et al. Autonomic changes during wake-sleep transition: a heart rate variability based approach. Auton Neurosci 2006;130(1–2):17–27.

65. Decker MJ, Eyal S, Shinar Z, et al. Validation of ECG-derived sleep architecture and ventilation in sleep apnea and chronic fatigue syndrome. Sleep Breath 2010;14(3):233–9.

66. Gorny SW, Allen RP, Krausman DT. Evaluation of an unattended monitoring system for automated detection of sleep apnea [abstract]. Sleep 2000;23(Suppl 2):A369.

67. Gorny SW, Spiro JR, Phillips B, et al. Initial findings from a multi-site evaluation of an unattended monitoring system for automatic detection of sleep disordered breathing events [abstract]. Sleep 2001;24(Suppl):A408.

68. Spiro JR, Gorry SW, Allen R, et al. Pilot evaluation of an ambulatory airflow pressure monitor for immediate identification of sleep disordered breathing events [abstract]. Sleep 2002;25(Suppl):A275.

69. de Almeida FR, Ayas NT, Otsuka R, et al. Nasal pressure recordings to detect obstructive sleep apnea. Sleep Breath 2006;10(2):62–9.

70. Grover SS, Pittman SD. Automated detection of sleep disordered breathing using a nasal pressure monitoring device. Sleep Breath 2008;12(4):339–45.

71. Pang KP, Gourin CG, Terris DJ. A comparison of polysomnography and the WatchPAT in the diagnosis of obstructive sleep apnea. Otolaryngol Head Neck Surg 2007;137(4):665–8.

72. Ayas NT, Pittman S, MacDonald M, et al. Assessment of a wrist-worn device in the detection of obstructive sleep apnea. Sleep Med 2003;4(5):435–42.

73. Pillar G, Bar A, Betito M, et al. An automatic ambulatory device for detection of AASM defined arousals from sleep: the WP100. Sleep Med 2003;4(3):207–12.

74. Bar A, Pillar G, Dvir I, et al. Evaluation of a portable device based on peripheral arterial tone for unattended sleep studies. Chest 2003;123(3):695–703.

75. Schnall RP, Shlitner A, Sheffy J, et al. Periodic, profound peripheral vasoconstriction—a new marker of obstructive sleep apnea. Sleep 1999; 22(7):939–46.

76. Pillar G, Malhotra A, Fogel R, et al. Detection of obstructive sleep disordered breathing events utilizing peripheral arterial tonometry and oximetry [abstract]. Sleep 2000;23(Suppl):1304.

77. Pittman S, Tal N, Pillar G, et al. Automatic detection of obstructive sleep-disordered breathing events using peripheral arterial tonometry and oximetry [abstract]. J Sleep Res 2000;9(Suppl 1):309.

78. O'Donnell CP, Allan L, Atkinson P, et al. The effect of upper airway obstruction and arousal on peripheral arterial tonometry in obstructive sleep apnea. Am J Respir Crit Care Med 2002;166(7):965–71.

79. Pillar G, Bar G, Shlitner A, et al. Autonomic Arousal Index (AAI): an automated detection based on peripheral arterial tonometry. Sleep 2002;25(5):541–7.

80. Zou D, Grote L, Peker Y, et al. Validation of a portable monitoring device for sleep apnea diagnosis in a population based cohort using synchronized home polysomnography. Sleep 2006;29(3): 367–74.

81. Hedner J, Pillar G, Pittman DS, et al. A novel adaptive wrist actigraphy algorithm for sleep-wake assessment in sleep apnea patients. Sleep 2004; 27(8):1560–6.

82. Herscovici S, Pe'er A, Papyan S, et al. Detecting REM sleep from the finger: an automatic REM sleep algorithm based on peripheral arterial tone (PAT) and actigraphy. Physiol Meas 2007;28(2):129–40.

83. Bresler M, Sheffy K, Pillar G, et al. Differentiating between light and deep sleep stages using an ambulatory device based on peripheral arterial tonometry. Physiol Meas 2008;29(5):571–84.

84. Pittman SD, Pillar G, Berry RB, et al. Follow-up assessment of CPAP efficacy in patients with obstructive sleep apnea using an ambulatory device based on peripheral arterial tonometry. Sleep Breath 2006;10(3):123–31.

85. Townsend D, Sharma A, Brauer E, et al. Assessing efficacy, outcomes, and cost savings for patients with obstructive sleep apnea using two diagnostic and treatment strategies. Sleep Diag Ther 2007; 1(7):1–8.

86. Berry RB, Hill G, Thompson L, et al. Portable monitoring and auto-titration versus polysomnography for the diagnosis and treatment of sleep apnea. Sleep 2008;31(10):1423–31.

87. Barrera JE, Holbrook AB, Santo J, et al. Pulse arterial tone and airway obstruction in sleep apnea [abstract]. Otolaryngol Head Neck Surg 2008; 139(Suppl 2):83.

88. Brinkley A, deWeerd AW. An investigation of reliability: nasal pressure and The SleepStrip [abstract]. J Sleep Res 2004;13(Suppl s1):97.

89. Shochat T, Hadas N, Molotsky A, et al. Validation of an apnea home screening device [abstract]. Eur Respir J 2004;3517. Available at: http://www.ers-education.org/pages/default.aspx?id=335&idBrowse= 19118&det=1. Accessed June 23, 2011.

90. Suvilehto J, Partinen M, Mikkola J, et al. The Sleep-Strip method as a screening tool for sleep apnea [abstract]. Sleep Med 2003;4(Suppl 1):210.

91. Leger D, Elbaz M, Stal V, et al. Evaluation of the "Sleep Strip," a simple device to screen apnea patients in the general population [abstract]. Sleep 2001;24(Suppl):A310.

92. Shochat T, Hadas N, Kerkhofs M, et al. The SleepStrip: an apnoea screener for the early detection of sleep apnoea syndrome. Eur Respir J 2002;19(1):121–6.

93. Garvey JF, Chua CP, Boyle P, et al. Home screening for obstructive sleep apnea syndrome using a combined holter-oximeter [abstract]. Am J Respir Crit Care Med 2009;179(Suppl):A2137.

94. Heneghan C, Chua CP, de Chazal P, et al. A home screening tool for obstructive sleep apnea using a combined holter-oximeter [abstract]. Am J Respir Crit Care Med 2007;175:A701.

95. Stern JC, Heneghan C, Shouldice R. Reliability of holter oximetry for home sleep apnea testing [abstract]. Otolaryngol Head Neck Surg 2008; 139(Suppl 2):83–4.

96. Stern JC, Shouldice R, Gold S, et al. A new device for home screening of obstructive sleep apnea using holter oximetry. Available at: http://www.nemon.com/ A%20New%20Device_Stern_et_al.pdf. Accessed March 1, 2011.

97. Claman D, Murr A, Tortter K. Clinical validation of the Bedbugg in detection of obstructive sleep apnea. Otolaryngol Head Neck Surg 2001;125(3):227–30.

98. Reichert JA, Bloch DA, Cundiff E, et al. Comparison of NovaSom QSG, a new sleep apnea home-diagnostic system, and polysomnography. Sleep Med 2003;4(3):213–8.

99. Kosseifi SG, Roy TM, Byrd RP, et al. Home sleep studies: the utility and referral pattern in a VA population [abstract]. Chest 2006;130(Suppl 4):263S–4S.

100. Durant KC, Kaufer L, Black J. Novel airflow sensor demonstrates linear relationship with pneumotachography [abstract]. Sleep 2003;26(Suppl):A267.

101. Stepnowsky CJ, Orr WC, Davidson TM. Nightly variability of sleep-disordered breathing measured over 3 nights. Otolaryngol Head Neck Surg 2004; 131(6):837–43.

102. Grover S, Bajwa I, Butchko AR, et al. A comparison of traditional laboratory-based polysomnography and the Alice PDx portable monitoring device, and the usability of the Alice PDx. Available at: http://www.healthcare.philips.com/asset.aspx?alt=& p=http://www.healthcare.philips.com/pwc_hc/main/ homehealth/sleep/alicepdx/PDF/alicepdx_White_ Paper_20091027.pdf. Accessed February 2, 2011.

103. Santos-Silva R, Sartori DE, Truksinas V, et al. Validation of a portable monitoring system for the diagnosis of obstructive sleep apnea syndrome. Sleep 2009;32(5):620–36.

104. Kuna ST, Seeger T, Brendel M. Intra-subject comparison of polysomnography and a type 3 potable monitor [abstract]. Sleep 2005;28(Suppl): 0956.

105. Wang Y, Teschler T, Weinreich G, et al. Validation of MicroMESAM as screening device for sleep disordered breathing. Pneumologie 2003;57(12):734–40 [in German].

106. Ragette R, Wang Y, Weinreich G, et al. Diagnostic performance of single airflow channel recording (ApneaLink) in home diagnosis of sleep apnea. Sleep Breath 2010;14(2):109–14.

107. Chen H, Lowe AA, Bai Y, et al. Evaluation of a portable recording device (ApneaLink) for case selection of obstructive sleep apnea. Sleep Breath 2010;13(3):213–9.

108. Vázquez JC, Tsai WH, Flemons WW, et al. Automated analysis of digital oximetry in the diagnosis of obstructive sleep apnoea. Thorax 2000;55(4): 302–7.

109. Michaelson PG, Allan P, Chaney J, et al. Validations of a portable home sleep study with twelve-lead polysomnography: comparisons and insights into a variable gold standard. Ann Otol Rhinol Laryngol 2006;115(11):802–9.

110. Dick R, Penzel T, Fietze I, et al. AASM standards of practice compliant validation of actigraphic sleep analysis from SOMNOwatch versus polysomnographic sleep diagnostics shows high conformity also among subjects with sleep disordered breathing. Physiol Meas 2010;31(12):1623–33.

111. Benes H, Küchler G, Kohnen R. Validation of the new actigraphy system SOMNOwatch for the measurement of periodic limb movements [abstract]. Sleep Med 2007;8(Suppl 1):P0062.

112. Hein H, Küchler G. Shifting of phase-angle for diagnostics of sleep-related breathing disorders. Presented at the 16th Annual Meeting of the German Sleep Society (DGSM). Kassel, October 16–18, 2008.

113. Herrmann M, Kercklow B, Kercklow K. Hypertonia and sleep apnea. Presented at the Internist Convention. Heringsdorf, 2004. Available at: http:// www.somnomedics-diagnostics.com/index.php? eID=tx_nawsecuredl&u=0&file=fileadmin/SOMNO medics/downloads/Publikationen/SOMNOscreen/ en/Hypertension_and_Sleep_Apnea_Internist_ Convention_2004.pdf&t=1308940830&hash= 34a9aa90d0dd4c4ef5e0021e5d7e5479. Accessed June 23, 2011.

114. Patzak A, Grosskurth D. A new method for noninvasive blood pressure measurement using pulse transition time. Presented at the 13th Annual Meeting of the German Sleep Society (DGSM). Berlin, October 13–15, 2005.

115. Dziewas R, Okegwo A, Waldmann N, et al. Pragmatic simplification of the visual sleep evaluation? Available at: http://www.somnomedics-diagnostics. com/index.php?eID=tx_nawsecuredl&u=0&file= fileadmin/SOMNOmedics/downloads/Publikationen/ SOMNOscreen/en/Validation_Kombi-Electrode.pdf&t= 1298525787&hash=5093f90dc1c9cad9f2641f84d269842f. Accessed February 22, 2011.

116. Krecklow B, Krecklow K, Zadeh A, et al. The significance of the phase angle analysis for the portrayal of sleep related breathing disorders that require treatment [abstract]. Pneumologie 2007;61(S1):P356.

117. Gesche H, Gosskurth D, Patzak A. A new method for noninvasive blood pressure measurement using pulse transition time. Presented at the International Congress Hypertension and the Kidney. Vienna, November 29–December 2, 2007.

118. Hein H, Warmuth R, Küchler G. Accuracy of the AASM-level 3 ambulatory monitoring device SOMNOscreen in unattended home measurements for sleep disordered breathing (SDB)? [abstract]. Sleep Med 2007;8(Suppl 1):P0064.

119. Tönnesmann U, Todtmoos RZ, Whehrawald K. Arousal-reaction and changes of body-position cause deviations of the 24h-RR-blood-pressure-records during sleep. Presented at the Annual Conference of the German Hypertension League. Bochum, November 21, 2007.

120. de Chazal P, Heneghan C, Sheridan E, et al. Automated processing of the single-lead electrocardiogram for the detection of obstructive sleep apnoea. IEEE Trans Biomed Eng 2003;50(6):686–96.

121. Moody GB, Mark RG, Zoccola A, et al. Derivation of respiratory signals from multi-lead ECGs. Comput Cardiol 1985;12:113–6.

122. Moody GB, Mark RG, Bump MA, et al. Clinical validation of the ECG-derived respiration (EDR) technique. Comput Cardiol 1986;13:507–10.

123. Penzel T, McNames J, Murray A, et al. Systematic comparison of different algorithms for apnoea detection based on electrocardiogram recordings. Med Biol Eng Comput 2002;40(4):402–7.

124. Bader G, Almersjö B. A comparison of sleep analysis according to polysomnography and to a sensor pad recording method [abstract]. Sleep 1999; 22(Suppl 1):C074.N.

125. Bader G, Kampe T, Tagdae T, et al. Descriptive physiological data on a sleep bruxism population. Sleep 1997;20(11):982–90.

126. Bader G. Prediction of drowsiness based on the study of the autonomic nervous system [abstract]. Sleep 2001;24(Suppl):A406.

127. Bader GG, Turesson K, Wallin A. Sleep-related breathing and movement disorders in healthy elderly and demented subjects. Dementia 1996;7(5):279–87.

128. Nerfeldt P, Nilsson B, Mayor L, et al. Weight reduction improves sleep, sleepiness, and metabolic status in obese sleep apnoea patients. Obes Res Clin Pract 2008;2(4):247–50.

129. Germain A, Hall M, Shear K, et al. Ecological study of sleep disruption in PTSD: a pilot study. Ann N Y Acad Sci 2006;1071:438–41.

130. Takeuchi T, Ogilvie RD, Murphy TI, et al. The relationship between REM sleep and intensive piano learning [abstract]. Sleep 2001;24(Suppl):A161.

131. Bader G. The transition from awakeness to drowsiness and sleep: a "micro-scoring" method to study hypnagogic EEG [abstract]. Sleep 2000; 23(Suppl 2):A372.

132. Bader G, Karlsson T, Sellersjö L. Movement-related variability of heart activity during sleep [abstract]. Sleep 2000;23(Suppl 2):A372.

133. van Selms MK, Lobbezoo F, Wicks DJ, et al. Craniomandibular pain, oral parafunctions, and psychological stress in a longitudinal case study. J Oral Rehabil 2004;31(8):738–45.

134. Bader G. A new scoring method to study hypnagogic EEG. Presented at the American Physiological Society Meeting on the Determinants of Vigilance: Interaction Between the Sleep and Circadian Systems. Fort Lauderdale, October 19–22, 1999.

135. Van der Zaag J, Lobbezoo F, Van der Avoort PG, et al. Effects of pergolide on severe sleep bruxism in a patient experiencing oral implant failure. J Oral Rehabil 2007;34(5):317–22.

136. Yucha CB, Tsai PS, Calderon KS. Ambulatory applications for monitoring physiological parameters. In: Zouridakis G, Moore J, editors. Biomedical technology and devices handbook. Boca Raton (FL): CRC Press; 2005. p. 27-1–27-23.

137. Bader G, Patterson S. Continuous glucose monitoring in subjects with insomnia [abstract]. Sleep 2006;29(Suppl):0770.

138. Bader G, Blomqvist C, Sellersjo L, et al. The Mozart/music effect in relaxation therapy: myth or neurophysiological evidence? [abstract]. J Sleep Res 2006;15(Suppl s1):P294.

139. Bader G, Eder DN. Elevating the head of the bed during sleep reduces snoring [abstract]. Sleep Med 2005;6(Suppl 2):P027.

140. Bader G. A pad for continuous topographic recording of body temperature [abstract]. J Sleep Res 2004;5(Suppl 1):41.

141. Bader G, Gillberg C, Johnson M, et al. Activity and sleep in children with ADHD [abstract]. Sleep 2003;26(Suppl):A136.

142. Bader G, Blomqvist C. The impact of bed firmness on sleep [abstract]. Sleep 2002;25(Suppl):A392.

143. Bader G, Blomqvist M, Kamper T. Motor activity during night sleep in patients with bruxism [abstract]. Presented at the 12th Annual Meeting of the Associated Professional Sleep Societies. New Orleans, June 18–23, 1998.

144. Bader G, Sillén U, Hjälmås K, et al. Nocturnal enuresis [abstract]. Presented at the 11th Annual Meeting of the Associated Professional Sleep Societies. San Francisco, June 10–15, 1997.

145. Nevéus T, Bader G, Sillén U. Enuresis, sleep, and desmopressin treatment. Acta Paediatr 2002; 91(10):1121–5.

146. Bader G, Nevéus T, Kruse S, et al. Sleep of primary enuretic children and controls. Sleep 2002;25(5):573–7.

147. Bader G, Lavigne G. Sleep bruxism: an overview of an oromandibular sleep movement disorder. Sleep Med Rev 2000;4(1):27–43.

148. Bader GG, Engdal S. The influence of bed firmness on sleep quality. Appl Ergon 2000;31(5):487–97.

149. Bader G, Kampe T, Tagdae T. Body movement during sleep in subjects with long-standing bruxing behavior. Int J Prosthodont 2000;13(4):327–33.

150. Westbrook PR, Levendowski DJ, Cvetinovic M, et al. Description and validation of the Apnea Risk Evaluation System: a novel method to diagnose sleep apnea-hypopnea in the home. Chest 2005;128(4):2166–75.

151. Ayappa I, Norman RG, Seelall V, et al. Validation of a self-applied unattended monitor for sleep disordered breathing. J Clin Sleep Med 2008;4(1):26–37.

152. Levendowski D, Steward D, Woodson BT, et al. The impact of obstructive sleep apnea variability measured in-lab versus in-home on sample size calculations. Int Arch Med 2009;2:2.

153. To KW, Chan WC, Chan TO, et al. Validation study of a portable monitoring device for identifying OSA in a symptomatic patient population. Respirology 2009;14(2):270–5.

154. Westbrook PR, Dickel MJ, Nicholson D, et al. Comparison of two limited-channel systems for the diagnosis of sleep apnea/hypopnea in the home. Sleep Diag Ther 2007;2(1):33–7.

155. Finkel KJ, Saager L, Safar-Zadeh E, et al. Obstructive sleep apnea: the silent pandemic [abstract]. Available at: http://www.watermarkmedical.com/publications/The_Silent_Pandemic_abstract.pdf. Accessed February 22, 2011.

156. Finkel KJ, Searleman AC, Tymkew H, et al. Prevalence of undiagnosed obstructive sleep apnea among surgical patients in an academic medical center. Sleep Med 2009;10(7):753–8.

157. Levendowski DJ, Morgan T, Montague J, et al. Prevalence of probable obstructive sleep apnea risk and severity in a population of dental patients. Sleep Breath 2008;12(4):303–9.

158. Levendowski DJ, Olmstead R, Popovic D, et al. Assessment of obstructive sleep apnea risk and severity in truck drivers: validation of a screening questionnaire. Sleep Diag Ther 2007;2(2):20–6.

159. Levendowski DJ, Rosen CL, Zavora T, et al. Feasibility of portable monitoring to detect obstructive sleep apnea in-home in adolescents: a pilot study [abstract]. Sleep 2008;31(Suppl):0188.

160. Levendowski D, Berka C, Popovic D, et al. Impact of age and position on severity of gender-specific sleep disordered breathing [abstract]. Sleep 2009;32(Suppl):0656.

161. Westbrook P, Levendowski DJ, Zavora T, et al. Night to night variability of in-home sleep studies—is one night enough? [abstract]. Sleep 2007;30(Suppl): 0555.

162. Rosenthal L, Dolan D. Comparison of subjective sleep position preference vs objective ambulatory data [abstract]. Sleep 2009;32(Suppl):1185.

163. Masdeu M, Hwang D, Mooney A, et al. Impact of clinical assessment on the difference between unattended limited monitoring and full in-lab PSG [abstract]. Sleep 2008;31(Suppl):0454.

164. Simmons M. Patient preferences comparing use of two home sleep testing devices [abstract]. Sleep Breath 2009;13(3):301–12, P12.

165. Popovic D, Levendowski DJ, Ayappa I, et al. Accuracy of automated sleep staging using signals from a single forehead site [abstract]. Sleep 2008; 31(Suppl):1007.

166. Popovic D, Velimirovic V, Ayappa I, et al. Sleep/wake classification using head actigraphy, snoring, and airflow signals [abstract]. Sleep 2009;32(Suppl): 1161.

167. Levendowski DJ, Morgan T, Melzer V, et al. Benefit of mandibular repositioning device therapy in patients with moderate and severe OSA [abstract]. Sleep 2009;32(Suppl):0621.

168. Popovic D, Morgan T, Montague J, et al. Impact of time on the treatment efficacy of mandibular positioning devices [abstract]. Sleep 2009;32(Suppl): 0620.

169. Westbrook P, Levendowski D, Henninger D, et al. Predicting effective continuous airway pressure (CPAP) based on laboratory titration and auto-titrating CPAP [abstract]. Sleep Med 2006;7(Suppl 2): P392.

170. Sasse S, Westbrook P, Levendowski D, et al. Accuracy of pulse oximetry during breath holding [abstract]. Presented at the American Thoracic Society International Conference. San Diego, May 20–25, 2005.

171. Popovic D, Morgan T, Melzer V, et al. Assessing changes in the apnea/hypopnea index resulting from increased vertical dimension of mandibular repositioning devices [abstract]. Sleep Breath 2009;13(3):P14.

172. Morgan T, Montague J, Melzer V, et al. Factors impacting mandibular-repositioning-device therapy at one-month [abstract]. Sleep Breath 2009;13(3):P15.

173. Levendowski D, Morgan T, Patrickus J, et al. Predicting changes in AHI resulting from mandibular repositioning device therapy [abstract]. Sleep Breath 2009;13(3):P16.

174. Morgan T, Popovic D, Melzer V, et al. Assessing change in AHI during a non-treatment washout period – Is there a halo effect? [abstract]. Sleep Breath 2009;13(3):P18.

175. Chung JW, Enciso R, Levendowski DJ, et al. Treatment outcomes of mandibular advancement devices in positional and nonpositional OSA patients. Oral Surg Oral Med Oral Pathol Oral Radiol Endod 2010;109(5):724–31.

Comparison of Portable Monitoring with Laboratory Polysomnography for Diagnosing Sleep-Related Breathing Disorders: Scoring and Interpretation

Max Hirshkowitz, PhD*, Amir Sharafkhaneh, MD, PhD

KEYWORDS

• Home sleep testing • Cardiopulmonary recording
• Sleep-related breathing disorder diagnosis
• Portable monitoring

Home sleep testing (HST) to diagnose sleep-disordered breathing is a reality that has been a long time coming. Long viewed as an anathema by purists and individuals strongly invested in laboratory polysomnography (PSG), HST arrives at a tumultuous time during health care transition. The arrival on the American scene, in some respects, appears sudden, even though various iterations and approaches date back 30 years, or more. Many sleep specialists were narrowly focused on laboratory PSG as the sleep diagnostic tool to use in conjunction with clinical assessment. Consequently, policies and procedures describe laboratory PSG in extraordinarily elaborate detail from specifics of recording to data summarization. However, it took 35 years before a single-source polysomnographic recording and scoring manual for sleep, central nervous system (CNS) arousals, sleep-related breathing, and sleep movement parameters was published with endorsement by a major clinical sleep society.[1]

The American Academy of Sleep Medicine (AASM) manual built on a foundation laid brick-by-brick by devoted clinicians and scientists fascinated by sleep and acutely aware that sleep disorders could disable patients emotionally and physically. The process of codifying procedures, validating them with science, and reaching consensus, took years. The groundwork preceding that processes took even longer. So, when Central Medicare Services (CMS) approved reimbursement for HST devices, approaches and techniques were suddenly propelled into the mainstream. Fortunately, general groundwork for classifying a wide assortment of HST devices had previously been laid. Nonetheless, proliferation of different biopotential and physiologic sensors and their possible factorial recombination in some cases defied existing classifications. Nonetheless, most HST devices fall into the level 3 classification that essentially represents a cardiopulmonary recorder.[2,3] The extent of validation for specific

Michael E. DeBakey VA Medical Center, Sleep Disorders & Research Center, Building 100, Room 6C-344, 2002 Holcombe Boulevard, Houston, TX 77030, USA
* Corresponding author.
E-mail address: maxh@bcm.edu

Sleep Med Clin 6 (2011) 283–292
doi:10.1016/j.jsmc.2011.05.004
1556-407X/11/$ – see front matter. Published by Elsevier Inc.

measurement approaches varied widely, ranging from proprietary manufacturers' test results to randomized controlled studies using standardized diagnostic criteria.

Faced with such diversity and an urgency to specify a guideline for recording, scoring, and interpretation, some guidance was needed. Rather than sink into paralysis induced by a complex morass, the solution was simple—borrow and slightly revise procedures from methodology already known well— in this case- laboratory PSG. But, HST using cardiopulmonary recorders and laboratory PSG differ in many ways. Differences include diagnostic criteria, signal recording, and disordered-breathing event scoring. Mere importation of rules and criteria from laboratory PSG to cardiopulmonary HST technique does not provide a good fit. Perhaps the greatest difference is in the overall interpretative approach.

PSG AND CARDIOPULMONARY RECORDER HST DIFFERENCES

Before addressing the multitude of details, it should be understood that a single core overarching difference between PSG and HST permeates all aspects of its existence and application. **PSG is a tool of discovery. HST is a tool of verification**. From the beginning, before Loomis and his cadre of scientist associates turned their focus to war effort-related applications, the first all-night sleep study was part of an intellectual exploration. Arguably, this first polysomnographic effort defined the process and patterns of the sleeping human brain.[4] Again, 25 years later, PSG was the tool of discovery with which Aserinsky unveiled rapid eye movement (REM) sleep.[5] And continuing to this day, many sleep disorders owe much of their discovery and validation to laboratory PSG (eg, obstructive sleep apnea, periodic limb movement disorder, REM sleep behavior disorder). By contrast, cardiopulmonary recorder HST's main purpose is to confirm sleep-disordered breathing. It does not even disconfirm (ie, rule-out) the diagnosis when test results are negative.

Diagnostic Criteria

Polysomnographic diagnostic criteria for sleep-related breathing disorder (SRBD) are expressed in terms of apnea, hypopnea, and respiratory effort-related arousal (RERA) frequencies. Episode frequency is normalized according to total sleep time to produce an index of the number of events per hour of sleep. Thus apnea index (AI), apnea+hypopnea index (AHI), and respiratory disturbance index (RDI, apnea+hypopnea+RERA) are calculated, and a patient exceeding threshold is

diagnosed. Currently AHI/RDI threshold is 15 (or more) events per hour in any patient (regardless of symptoms or comorbid conditions) or 5 (or more) events in a patient with symptoms or a comorbid condition usually associated with SRBD. By contrast, cardiovascular recorder HST results only yield AI and AHI but not RDI, because RERA cannot be scored without a technique for detecting CNS arousals. Thus, unless the patient has many complete cessations of breathing (apnea episodes), readily desaturates (which may represent prolonged breathing events and/or comorbid lung problems), or both, diagnostic criteria are less likely to be met. Furthermore, the denominator for indices is, by necessity, total recording time rather than total sleep time, because sleep is not discerned by cardiopulmonary recorders. Thus, the cardiopulmonary HSTs are less sensitive than laboratory PSGs on 2 counts and have higher false-negative liability. Consequently, HST is only recommended in patients for whom there is already a high clinical suspicion of SRBD. HST can rule-in but not rule-out sleep-disordered breathing. Thus, contrary to popular parlance, HST is not a screening test (ie, a test applied to non-symptomatic populations like purified protein derivative (PPD) skin test for tuberculosis).

Signal Recording

Polysomnographic channels used for routine clinical evaluations are generally well standardized with amplification, recording, and display techniques mostly pecified. By contrast, HST signals are diverse and sometimes poorly validated. The specific recording details may be undisclosed, sometimes intentionally for proprietary reasons. In preparation for laboratory PSG, a trained technologist attaches, tests, and calibrates monitoring devices. By contrast, patients undergoing HST usually self-apply sensors, and no calibration procedure is performed. The technologist's presence during attended laboratory procedures helps assure recording continuity and documentation of interruptions, incidents, or issues arising during the recording. HSTs progress without any expectation of intervention or accurate documentation. If a sensor detaches, it will likely remain detached. If the patient awakens and turns on the television, there may be no way for the clinician reviewing the HST to know.

Disordered-Breathing Event Scoring

Both laboratory PSG and cardiopulmonary recorder HST seek to identify and classify sleep-disordered breathing events. As previously mentioned, 1 big difference between the procedures is cardiopulmonary HST's not having facility to score CNS arousal.

Some recorders include frontal or hairline EEG; however, the utility for scoring CNS arousal from this derivation is not validated. PSG scoring rules for CNS arousals specifically indicate occipital scalp derivations, because decades of topographic comparisons indicate it is the most sensitive locus.[6] There is little debate concerning whether complete airway occlusion represents a pathophysiological event. By contrast, the metric for and consequence of partial obstructions limiting airflow (hypopnea) have been controversial topics for years. In essence, a hypopnea is merely a shallow breath and is not intrinsically pathophysiological. However, when it is associated with significant oxyhemoglobin desaturations or it disturbs sleep, then the breathing event becomes clinically meaningful-not for what it is but rather the consequences it produces. Without ability to score CNS arousals, cardiopulmonary HST can only identify hypopnea leading to oxyhemoglobin desaturations. Thus, the RDI, which includes episodes of reduced airflow provoking arousal, cannot be calculated. To make matters worse, if the oximetry channel detaches or malfunctions (which in the authors' experience is the most common HST signal failure), then even hypopnea cannot be scored, making outcome solely dependent on apnea episode frequency.

The AASM laboratory PSG operational definition for a sleep apnea episode requires a 10-second (or longer) 90% drop (or greater) in the nasal/oral airflow channel's peak-to-trough amplitude persisting for at least 90% of the event's duration.[1] Each apnea episode is further classified as central, obstructive, or mixed. This classification indicates whether respiratory effort is absent throughout, present throughout, or present only during part of the episode. The recommended operational definition for hypopnea requires a greater than or equal to 10-second, greater than or equal to 30%-drop in nasal pressure signal amplitude (compared with baseline) persisting for at least 90% of the event's duration and associated with a greater than or equal to 4% drop in oxygen saturation. No such detailed definitions exist for HST. Part of the problem is the great diversity in the sensors and parameters embedded in HST recording systems (**Table 1**), making it very difficult to standardize specific rules. Scoring basically relies on pattern recognition, largely based on threshold values or amplitude variation patterns.

Table 1
Measurement parameters and approaches used by home sleep testing devices

Parameter	Measurement Approach
Sleep	Traditional scalp electrode
	Central forehead or hairline electrode
	Actigraphy
	Pulse volume variability
Airflow	Nasal pressure
	Nasal–oral temperature
	Breath sounds
	Surrogate with tonometry
	Surrogate with cardiopulmonary index
Respiratory Effort	Ribcage and/or abdominal movement
	Snoring sounds
	Inductive pheythesmography
	Stretch or strain gauges
	Static charge sensitive bed
Oximetry	Ear, finger, or forehead probe

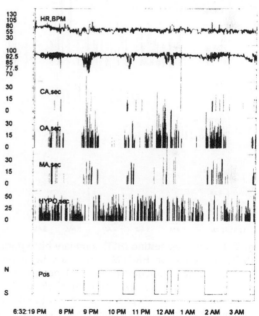

Fig. 1. Home sleep testing (HST) summary histogram. Activity is present on HR-BPM (heart rate–beats per minute), SpO2 (oxyhemoglobin saturation percentage), CA (central-type apnea), OA (obstructive apnea), MA (mixed apnea), HYPO (hypopnea), and Pos (position- S [supine] and N [nonsupine]) channels. A clear pattern of sleep apnea and hypopnea is visible. Prominent desaturations recurred approximately every 90 minutes and may have derived from REM, supine body position, or both; however, without sleep staging, this hypothesis cannot be verified. Overall AHI was 66.6; SpO2 nadir was 71%, and the patient spent 12.5 minutes with oxyhemoglobin below 85%.

While most HST recorders include automated scoring commonly used to calculate the primary clinical outcome measures, PSGs are largely scored and reviewed manually by trained polysomnographic technologists. Perhaps the most important, but unstated, element in PSG scoring is artifact recognition using the diverse activity patterns in any of the recording channels. By viewing simultaneously airflow, nasal pressure, rib cage movement, abdominal movement, intercostal electromyographic activity, multiple electroencephalographic channels, electrooculograms, snoring sounds, oximetry, heart rhythm, leg movement, and body position, the technologist has a wealth of information to infer body movements, sweating, coughing, teeth grinding, blinking,

talking, and other activities that can contaminate the breathing sensor outputs. The paucity of information available on HST recordings can leave one scratching his or her head wondering what the signal pattern means. Nonetheless, a reduced set of signal pattern recognition strategies ultimately is used by the clinician when interpreting HST results.

PRACTICAL APPROACH FOR HST INTERPRETATION

HST interpretation begins with a single question... "Does this patient have a clinically significant sleep related breathing disorder?" To answer that question the clinician must first evaluate the HST recording's technical quality to determine if it is good enough to answer the question. HSTs are recorded in the field, in uncontrolled environments, with hookups performed by minimally trained individuals (the patient, who may be already impaired

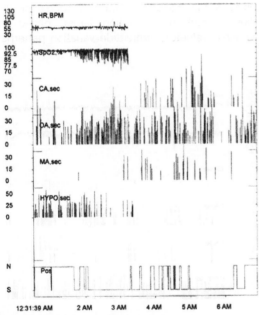

Fig. 2. Home sleep testing (HST) summary histogram. Activity is present on HR-BPM (heart rate–beats per minute), SpO2 (oxyhemoglobin saturation percentage), CA (central-type apnea), OA (obstructive apnea), MA (mixed apnea); HYPO (hypopnea), and Pos (position-S [supine] and N [nonsupine]) channels. A clear pattern of sleep apnea and hypopnea is visible. Note that the SpO2 channel malfunctions approximately halfway through the recording, and therefore no additional hypopnea episodes are scored. Because this patient had severe sleep-disordered breathing, AHI (even missing all possible hypopnea in the second half of recording) was still 52.8; SpO2 nadir was 60%, and the patient spent 7.5 minutes with SpO2 below 85% (that could be documented before the sensor malfunctioned). As is often the case with unattended HST recordings, once the SpO2 probe became nonfunctional (probably becoming detached), it remained so for the rest of the recording.

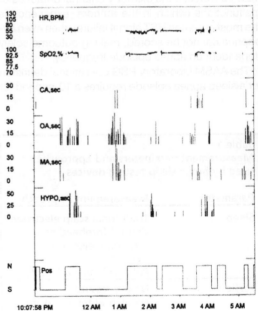

Fig. 3. Home sleep testing (HST) summary histogram. Activity is present on HR-BPM (heart rate–beats per minute), SpO2 (oxyhemoglobin saturation percentage), CA (central-type apnea), OA (obstructive apnea), MA (mixed apnea), HYPO (hypopnea), and Pos (position-S [supine] and N [nonsupine]) channels. An intermittent pattern of sleep apnea and hypopnea is visible; however, the SpO2 channel malfunctions at irregular intervals, thereby limiting the number of hypopnea episodes that can be scored. In total, this patient had an AHI of 16.8 with a recorded SpO2 nadir of 88%. The time spent with SpO2 below 85% is 0; however, that statistic may be misleading, because the channel recording was unreliable and intermittent.

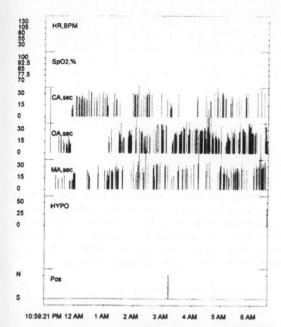

Fig. 4. Home sleep testing (HST) summary histogram. Activity is present on HR-BPM (heart rate–beats per minute), CA (central-type apnea), OA (obstructive apnea), MA (mixed apnea), HYPO (hypopnea), and Pos (position- S [supine] and N [nonsupine]) channels. A clear pattern of sleep apnea episodes is visible. Note that the SpO2 channel did not record at any time during this HST; therefore no hypopnea episodes were scored. Because this patient had severe sleep-disordered breathing, rife with apneas, AHI (even missing all possible hypopnea) was still 58.2. No SpO2 nadir or time spent with SpO2 below 85% could be calculated.

by his or her condition), with little or no documentation about events concurrent with the actual procedure. Timing of testing will vary widely test durations will fluctuate, and devices will malfunction. Sensors also will detach. The good news is that there are few ways these problems will produce false-positive test results. The bad news is that all of these problems can decrease test sensitivity and produce false-negative tests results. The 1 mitigating factor concerning false-negative test result problem is that the patient being tested (if properly referred) will have a high clinical suspicion for sleep-disordered breathing such that even a sensitivity-compromised test will confirm diagnosis.

The clinician begins by reviewing the overall nightly histogram and the raw data tracings to evaluate technical quality (recording and scoring). Event scoring largely depends on the recording's technical quality. The immediate goal is to verify the sleep-disordered breathing event scoring. Once the clinician determines his or her level of agreement with the scoring, evaluation is ultimately reduced to 3 options. The HST recording's technical quality may be (1) inadequate to make a diagnosis, (2) compromised but adequate to diagnose some form of sleep-disordered breathing, or (3) good, clearly indicating obstructive, central, or complex sleep apnea. The clinician's first task is to rule-in or rule-out option one. The second task can be much more difficult; that is, to determine diagnostic confidence level based on the recordings technical quality. In the process of reviewing their first 5000 HSTs, the authors

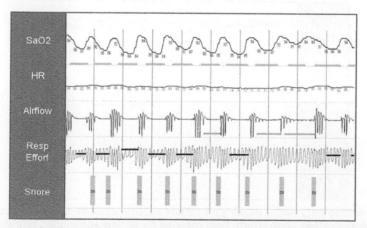

Fig. 5. Home sleep testing (HST) tracing showing a 5-minute epoch with oxyhemoglobin saturation (SaO2), heart rate (HR), airflow, respiratory effort (Resp Effort), and snoring sounds (Snore). This illustration clearly shows obstructive sleep apnea episodes with prominent oxyhemoglobin desaturation events.

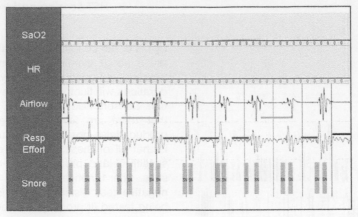

Fig. 6. Home sleep testing (HST) tracing showing a 5-minute epoch with airflow, respiratory effort (Resp Effort), and snoring sounds (Snore). Data channels for oxyhemoglobin saturation (SaO2) and heart rate (HR) are nonfunctional. Nonetheless, apnea is clearly present and periodic. Although respiratory effort channel is functioning poorly, snore sound channel activity testify to the probable obstructive nature of these apnea events. Furthermore, because sleep-disordered breathing events are apneas, they can be scored without SaO2; if they were hypopnea, Central Medicare Services (CMS) scoring criteria would not be met due to SaO2's absence.

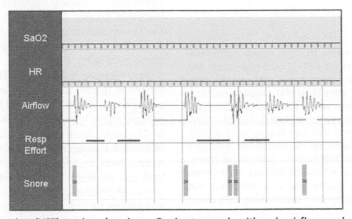

Fig. 7. Home sleep testing (HST) tracing showing a 5-minute epoch with only airflow and snoring sounds. Data channels for oxyhemoglobin saturation (SaO2), heart rate (HR), and respiratory effort (Resp Effort) are nonfunctional. It should be noted that apnea events are clearly discernable; however, their classification as central or obstructive is uncertain. Snore sound channel activity suggests the first, fourth, fifth, and seventh episodes are obstructive.

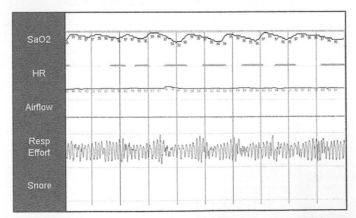

Fig. 8. Home sleep testing (HST) tracing showing a 5-minute epoch with oxyhemoglobin saturation (SaO2), heart rate (HR), and respiratory effort (Resp Effort). Data channels for airflow and snoring sounds are nonfunctional. There appear to be periodic sleep-disordered breathing events (based on repeated oxyhemoglobin desaturations coupled with waxing and waning respiratory effort). However, the type, classification as central or obstructive, and certainty of these events are unknown.

Table 2
iScore grading scheme for cardiopulmonary home sleep testing recordings

| | Data Recorder Channels | | | | |
| | Air Flow | SaO2 | Respiratory Effort | Snore Sounds | |
iScore					Interpretability Statement
10	x	x	x	x	Pattern can diagnose obstructive or central SRBD
	x	x	x	—	Pattern can diagnose obstructive or central SRBD
9	x	x	—	x	Pattern can diagnose SRBD of unknown type[a]
	x	x	—	—	Pattern can diagnose SRBD of unknown type
8	x	—	x	x	Pattern can diagnose obstructive or central SRBD if there are a sufficient number of apnea episodes[b]
	x	—	x	—	Pattern can diagnose obstructive or central SRBD if there are a sufficient number of apnea episodes[b]
7	x	—	—	x	Pattern can diagnose SRBD of unknown type if there are a sufficient number of apnea episodes[b] Snoring may help identify obstructive apnea episodes
6	x	—	—	—	Pattern can diagnose SRBD of unknown type if there are a sufficient number of apnea episodes[b]
5	—	x	x	x	Pattern may strongly suggest (but not diagnose) obstructive or central SRBD
	—	x	x	—	Pattern may strongly suggest (but not diagnose) obstructive or central SRBD[c]
4	—	x	—	x	Pattern may strongly suggest (but not diagnose) SRBD of unknown type[d]
3	—	x	—	—	Pattern may strongly suggest (but not diagnose) SRBD of unknown type
2	—	—	x	x	Pattern may weakly suggest (but not diagnose) possible central or obstructive SRBD
1	—	—	x	—	Pattern may weakly suggest (but not diagnose) central SRBD[e]
0	—	—	—	x	Not interpretable

Abbreviations: iScore, interpretability score; SaO2, oxygen saturation; SRBD, sleep related breathing disorder.

[a] Snoring can sometimes serves as surrogate for effort when hypopnea episodes are occurring (ie, increased resistance producing vibration), allowing diagnosis of obstructive SRBD.

[b] Hypopnea episodes may be suggested but are unconfirmed, thereby, increasing the chance of a false-negative study.

[c] When both effort and SaO2 drop, it is likely that an event of unknown type has occurred; if effort drops, but SaO2 does not, then there may be a central apnea episode. If SaO2 drops, but effort does not, then an obstructive event has likely occurred. Ultimately, even though some events are identifiable, the proportion of central to obstructive cannot be determined; consequently, diagnosis cannot be determined.

[d] Snoring, as a surrogate measure of respiratory effort, can potentially identify SRBD events as obstructive.

[e] An important limitation is that the pattern can potentially identify only central apnea episodes.

developed 2 conceptual tools to assist in this endeavor: (1) an interpretability score and (2) a margin of error scale.

Interpretability Score (iScore)

HST technical problems invariably generate missing data. In some sense, the HST is a PSG with missing data (missing sleep, leg movements, and some respiratory signals). It is already known that partial data can sometimes tell a story, albeit sometimes a partial story. The key data for

Table 3
Margin of errors for AHI (or AHI corrected by interpretability index)

AHI	Margin of Error
0–15	Does not meet diagnostic criteria
>15–20	High margin of error possible
>20–30	Moderate margin of error possible
>30	Low margin of error

Table 4
Parameter definitions and variable identifiers for final report

General Category	Parameter	Variable Identifier
Identifiers	Primary	PTFULLNAME
	Secondary	PTSSSNLAST4
Recording and patient information	Date of study	STUDYDATE
	Patient's age	AGE
	Patient's sex	SEX
	Patient's body mass index	BMI
	Epworth Sleepiness Scale score	ESS
	CMS comorbidity indicator[a]	CMSRFI
Elemental data points	Duration of recording (minutes)	TIMEINBED
	Number of central apneas	NCENTRALS
	Number of obstructive apnea	NOBSTRUCTS
	Number of mixed apnea	NMIXED
	Number of hypopnea	NHYPOP
	Number of minutes SaO2 was below 85%	M02LT85
	SaO2 nadir during the recording	O2NADIR
Indexed parameters (derived data)	Apnea index	AI
	Central apnea index	CAI
	Apnea + hypopnea index	AHI
	SRBD classification as mild, moderate, or severe	SRBDSVRTY
Clinician entered technical comments on study	Primary Technical Comment (code as):	TECHNICALCOMMENT1
	1. Technical quality of HST is insufficient to make interpretation	
	2. Technical quality of HST is compromised but available data show SRBD pattern	
	3. Technical quality of HST is good, and data show SRBD pattern	
	Secondary technical comment (free form)	TECHNICALCOMMENT2
Clinical outcome determination	Possible Clinical Outcomes (code as):	SRBDOUTCOME
	1. Patient has obstructive SRBD and is candidate for CPAP titration	
	2. Patient has obstructive SRBD and is candidate for CPAP titration or oral appliance	
	3. Patient has central SRBD and may need BPAP, ASV, or AVAPS	
	4. Patient has complex SRBD and may need ASV	
	5. Patient has undetermined type of SRBD and is a possible candidate for CPAP or BPAP titration	
	6. Recording not interpretable due to technical problems- order laboratory PSG or try HST again	
	7. Recording is too short- there is not enough data to make diagnosis- order PSG or try HST again	
	8. Patient did not meet diagnostic threshold- order laboratory PSG	
	SaO2 Determination (code as):	SAO2OUTCOME
	1. Patient should be referred to determine need for supplemental O2 (note- this is for referral now rather than later)	
	2. Patient should be referred to determine need for supplemental O2 if it does not normalize with PAP	

Abbreviations: ASV, adaptive servoventilation; AVAPS, average volume assured pressure support; BPAP, bilevel positive airway pressure; CMS, Central Medicare Services; CPAP, continuous positive airway pressure; HST, home sleep therapy; SRBD, sleep-related breathing disorder.

[a] CMS Comorbidity indicator. Does patient have hypertension, heart disease, mood disorder, cognitive impairment, insomnia, or history of stroke? If yes, code CMSRFI as 1; otherwise code as 0.

detecting sleep-disordered breathing events recorded by cardiopulmonary HST devices include airflow, respiratory effort, oxyhemoglobin saturation level, and snoring sounds. Review of the overall nightly histogram quickly provides the reviewer with global impressions and efficiently unveils missing or intermittently functional data channels (**Figs. 1–4**). Raw data tracings show more detailed patterns from which sleep-disordered breathing events can be discerned and validated (**Figs. 5–8**). **Table 2** shows the interpretability grading schema the authors developed for cardiopulmonary HST recordings.

Interpretability of a specified time domain segment derives from which recording channels are functioning and activity present within those channels. Overall interpretability is calculated by averaging hourly iScores (highest score for half (or more) minutes of each hour) and expressed as a fraction (ie, divided 10). The iScore can then be multiplied by the severity index to estimate certainty of diagnosis by creating a corrected AHI for consideration against the margin of error. For example, a 7.2-hour HST with hourly segment iScores of 10, 10, 10, 8, 8, 7, and 2 has an average iScore of 0.786 (or roughly 78.6% interpretable).

Margin of Error Scale

It stands to reason that technically adequate HST recordings revealing high AHIs (eg, 60 events per hour—4 times greater than diagnostic criteria) have a low margin of error. By contrast, HSTs finding AHI near diagnostic threshold have an intrinsically higher margin of error and inspire less confidence in the result. By reviewing computer logs, the authors found an inverse correlation between confidence in the result and the time spent reviewing HSTs for interpretation. Interpretive review duration reached a stable minimum on records with AHI greater than 30 events per hour (approximately an order of magnitude above the diagnostic threshold). Interestingly, the time function was not linear. Incrementally more time was spent as the overall AHI neared diagnostic threshold; however, the authors were unable to calculate the exact function. Therefore, they somewhat arbitrarily set margin of error scale points at values shown on **Table 3**.

Thus, in the previous example where the calculated iScore was 0.786, if the HST had an AHI of 25.1, the certainty estimate would reduce an AHI to 19.7, which falls within the high margin of error category. Such a recording might be deemed

Table 5 Sample report template for home sleep test	
Paragraph	**Text**
1	PTFULLNAME was referred for evaluation of sleep related breathing disorders. Sleep evaluation was performed on STUDYDATE using a HSTNAME&MODEL portable cardiopulmonary recorder [CPT code 95806]. The sleep specialist reviewing and interpreting this recording made the following comment: TECHNICALCOMMENT1 & TECHNICALCOMMENT2. During the TIMEINBED minutes of recording, there were NCENTRALS central apnea, NOBSTRUCTS obstructive apnea, NMIXED mixed apnea, and NHYPOP episodes of hypopnea. Apnea + hypopnea index was AHI and the lowest oxygen level recorded was O2NADIR. IF MO2LT85>1 THEN Additionally, the patient spent MO2LT85 minutes below 85 percent oxygen saturation.
2	<At this point in the report include SRBDOUTCOME, SAO2OUTCOME and other clinical comments or text>
3	In the meanwhile, the patient should be cautioned about the use of central nervous system depressants near bedtime (especially alcohol, sedatives, and hypnotics) because they may further impair sleep-related breathing. It is also critically important that patients with sleep disorders attain and maintain an adequate sleep schedule (a minimum of 7.5–8.0 hours in bed per night) because sleep deprivation exacerbate most sleep pathologies and is a major contributor to sleepiness and/or fatigue. IF BMI>40 THEN "Patient should lose weight with medical supervision." IF BMI BETWEEN 30 AND 40 THEN "Patient should attain and maintain ideal body weight." IF PATIENT HAS SRBD THEN "Patient should be cautioned to avoid sedative hypnotics or alcohol near bedtime because they can worsen the sleep related breathing disorder." Finally, we advise the patient to avoid driving or operating heavy equipment when sleepy or fatigued.

Abbreviation: CPT, current procedural terminology.

compromised but adequate to diagnose some form of sleep-disordered breathing. Certainly an HST with an iScore-corrected AHI less than 20 would require much more careful review to finalize diagnosis than one with an AHI of 58.9 (whose iScore-corrected AHI was 46.3). The latter record would fall in the low margin of error category; therefore, confidence would be high.

THE HST REPORT

Once the technical evaluation is complete; the parameters have been validated, and the confidence in the result established, then the overarching primary question can be answered. In other words... does the test confirm a SRBD diagnosis? The cardiopulmonary HST can verify or fail to verify. A failure to verify diagnosis does not ensure the patient does not have sleep-disordered breathing. Failure on HST should be followed with laboratory PSG, which is a much more sensitive test. HST possible outcomes include

> The patient has either obstructive, central, or an undetermined-type of SRBD
> The patient is a candidate for continuous, bilevel, or auto-titrating positive airway pressure (CPAP, BPAP, or APAP, respectively), adaptive servoventilation, or average volume pressure support titration or an oral appliance
> The recording is not interpretable due to technical problems or inadequate duration
> The patient did not meet diagnostic threshold, and a laboratory PSG is required.

Secondarily, the patient may need to be referred to determine if nocturnal supplemental O2 is needed. As is routine with final reports based on PSG, a host of good clinical practice statements should be included concerning maintaining an adequate sleep schedule, avoiding sedating medication or alcohol proximal to bed time, weight control (if appropriate), and caution against driving or engaging in potentially dangerous activities when sleepy or fatigued. **Tables 4** and **5** provide a sample listing of the parameters needed for an HST report and a simple format for reporting.

SUMMARY

Cardiopulmonary HST devices are tools of verification for diagnosing sleep-related breathing disorders. They can rule-in but not rule-out diagnosis. Types, channels, capabilities, and validation vary widely. Overall recording technique, scoring practices, the types of problems encountered, and interpretation strategies for cardiopulmonary recorders differ greatly from those used in traditional sleep studies. Diagnostic sensitivity with HST is lower than that for PSG, largely due to data limitations. Nonetheless, the shortcomings are usually offset by performing home sleep tests only on patients with high pretest probabilities for sleep-disordered breathing. This article also discussed using an interpretability score and a margin of error scale as techniques to index confidence in clinical interpretive outcomes. Finally, a template for reporting portable monitoring results was included (see **Table 5**).

REFERENCES

1. Iber C, Ancoli-Israel S, Chesson A, et al. The AASM manual for the scoring of sleep and associated events: rules, terminology, and technical specifications. 1st edition. Westchester (IL): American Academy of Sleep Medicine; 2007.
2. Chesson AL, Berry RB, Pack A. Practice parameters for the use of portable monitoring devices in the investigation of suspected obstructive sleep apnea in adults. Sleep 2003;26:907–13.
3. Collop NA, Anderson WM, Boehlecke B, et al. Clinical guidelines for the use of unattended portable monitors in the diagnosis of obstructive sleep apnea in adult patients. J Clin Sleep Med 2007;3:737–47.
4. Loomis AL, Harvey N, Hobart GA. Cerebral states during sleep, as studied by human brain potentials. J Exp Psychol 1937;21:127–44.
5. Aserinsky E, Kleitman N. Regularly occurring periods of eye motility, and concomitant phenomena. Science 1953;118:273–4.
6. Bonnet M, Carley D, Carskadon M, et al. EEG arousals: scoring rules and examples Sleep 1992; 15:173–84

Outcome Measures for Assessing Portable Monitor Testing for Sleep Apnea

Samuel T. Kuna, MD[a,b,*]

KEYWORDS

- Polysomnogram • Apnea-hypopnea index
- Cost-effectiveness

Obstructive sleep apnea (OSA) is a major public health issue. Population-based epidemiologic studies estimate the prevalence of sleep apnea/hypopnea syndrome (apnea-hypopnea index [AHI]>5 events/h with excessive daytime sleepiness) at 2% of adult women and 4% of adult men in the US population. A substantial proportion of these individuals are undiagnosed.[1–3] Existing evidence suggests that OSA is an independent risk factor for motor vehicle accidents, neurocognitive deficits, and cardiovascular morbidity and mortality.[4,5] Evidence also indicates that appropriate treatment of OSA reduces the risk of these consequences.[6–9] However, the need to perform costly and labor-intensive polysomnography (PSG) in a sleep laboratory limits patient access to diagnosis and treatment.[10,11] Relatively inexpensive, commercially available, and portable monitors might facilitate earlier recognition of OSA and faster initiation of treatment, thereby reducing its health care burden.[12–17] Interest in the clinical application of portable monitor devices is growing rapidly, and being used as a mainstay approach to the management of OSA in some settings. In 2007, the Agency for Healthcare Research and Quality issued an evidence-based review on portable monitor testing.[18] Despite the intuitive appeal of portable monitor testing, high-quality empiric evidence concerning their role in the clinical management of patients with sleep apnea is limited. Consequently, portable monitors have failed to gain widespread acceptance in sleep medicine.

EVIDENCE-BASED REVIEWS OF PORTABLE MONITORS FOR DIAGNOSIS OF OSA

The use of portable monitors for the diagnosis of patients with OSA remains controversial. In 2007, a task force of the American Academy of Sleep Medicine (AASM) issued the following clinical guidelines for the use of unattended portable monitors for the diagnosis of OSA in adults.[13]

1. Unattended portable monitoring should be performed only in conjunction with a comprehensive history and physical examination.
2. Portable monitor testing may be used as an alternative to PSG for the diagnosis of OSA in patients with a high pretest probability of moderate to severe OSA but is not appropriate for the diagnosis of OSA in patients with significant comorbid medical conditions.
3. Portable monitor testing is not appropriate for the diagnostic evaluation of patients suspected of having comorbid sleep disorders.

This work was supported by Grant No. IIR 02-041-2 from the VHA Health Services Research and Development and the Center for Health Equity Research and Promotion at the Philadelphia VA Medical Center.
Author Disclosure: Respironics, Inc: Contract including salary support - Investigator in a clinical research studies and Respironics, Inc: Equipment loaned for NIH and VA funded research studies.
a Pulmonary, Critical Care and Sleep Medicine, Philadelphia VA Medical Center, 3900 Woodland Avenue (111P), Philadelphia, PA 19104, USA
b University of Pennsylvania School of Medicine, 3400 Spruce Street, Philadelphia, PA 19104, USA
* Pulmonary, Critical Care and Sleep Medicine, Philadelphia VA Medical Center, 3900 Woodland Avenue (111P), Philadelphia, PA 19104.
E-mail address: skuna@mail.med.upenn.edu

Sleep Med Clin 6 (2011) 293–307
doi:10.1016/j.jsmc.2011.05.005
1556-407X/11/$ – see front matter. Published by Elsevier Inc.

4. Portable monitor testing is not appropriate for the general screening of asymptomatic populations.
5. Portable monitor testing may be indicated for the diagnosis of OSA in patients for whom in-laboratory PSG is not possible by virtue of immobility, safety, or critical illness.
6. Portable monitor testing may also be indicated to monitor the response to noncontinuous positive airway pressure treatments for sleep apnea.
7. The portable monitor device must allow for display of raw data with the capability of manual scoring or editing of automated scoring by a qualified sleep technician/technologist.

These clinical guidelines were based on the evidence-based medicine available to the task force and are likely to require modification as new evidence in this rapidly evolving field becomes available.

Portable monitors are intended primarily for unattended home recordings, but they can be used under either attended or unattended conditions and in a variety of locations, including the sleep laboratory and health care facilities (eg, to perform tests on hospitalized patients). Numerous portable monitors for the diagnosis of OSA are commercially available. In 1994, a task force on portable monitor testing created by the American Sleep Disorders Association (the current AASM) classified 4 different levels of sleep testing (**Table 1**).[19] The type 1 test is attended PSG performed in a sleep laboratory. Testing with portable monitors is categorized as types 2 to 4 based on the number and type of signal recorded. However, monitors within a given category may vary widely with regard to the signals recorded, the sensors used to record the signals, and processing of the signals.

TYPE 2 PORTABLE MONITORS

Type 2 portable monitors can record the same signals as in-laboratory diagnostic PSG. Type 2 monitors are unlikely to gain widespread clinical application because the need to attach the bipolar sensors for sleep staging usually requires a technologist to travel to the patient's home. However, type 2 monitors have proved useful in clinical research.[20–23] The type 2 monitors eliminate the need of investigators to compete with clinicians for access to overnight testing in a clinical sleep center, allowing greater flexibility in scheduling research studies within fixed protocol timelines. The ability to perform PSG at home also decreases burden on the research participants. In multicenter studies, the use of a type 2 monitor in multicenter studies standardizes PSG data collection across clinical sites that differ in the computer data collection systems used to record their in-laboratory studies. Standards for using type 2 monitors in clinical research studies were established by the Sleep Heart Health Study.[22] In that cross-sectional multicenter study of more than 6000 participants, technologists visited the participants' homes in the evening to attach the sensors and returned the next morning to retrieve the equipment. Rigorous training, certification, and quality control measures resulted in a less than 8% overall failure rate. Similar failure rates for home unattended type 2 monitor recordings have been reported by another multicenter study, Sleep AHEAD (Action for Health in Diabetes).[21]

TYPE 3 AND TYPE 4 PORTABLE MONITORS

Home unattended studies with type 3 and type 4 monitors are used primarily to evaluate patients

Table 1
Current classification of the different types of sleep studies

Sleep Test	Description	Personnel	Minimum Signals Required
Type 1	PSG performed in a sleep laboratory	Attended	Minimum of 7 signals, including EEG, EOG, chin EMG, ECG, airflow, respiratory effort and oxygen saturation
Type 2	Portable PSG	Unattended	Same as type 1
Type 3	Portable testing limited to sleep apnea	Attended and unattended	Minimum of 4 signals, including ECG or heart rate, oxygen saturation, and at least 2 channels of respiratory movement, or respiratory movement and airflow
Type 4	Continuous recording of 1 or more signals	Unattended	Usually pulse oximetry

Abbreviations: ECG, electrocardiogram; EEG, electroencephalogram; EMG, electromyogram; EOG, electrooculography.
Data from Ferber R, Millman RP, Coppola M, et al. Portable recording in the assessment of obstructive sleep apnea: ASDA standards of practice. Sleep 1994;17:378–92.

for the diagnosis of sleep apnea, determine the efficacy of positive airway pressure and oral appliance treatment, and assess the adequacy of arterial oxygen saturation during the sleep period. Type 3 portable monitors record a minimum of 4 signals, including electrocardiogram or heart rate, oxygen saturation, and at least 2 channels of respiratory movement, or respiratory movement and airflow. Almost all type 4 portable monitors record oxygen saturation by pulse oximetry with 1 or more additional signals. In the United States, the Center for Medicare and Medicaid Services requires that type 4 recordings have at least 3 channels. Depending on the signals recorded, type 4 monitors may not be able to detect sleep disordered breathing that is not associated with oxygen desaturation and they are generally unable to distinguish central from obstructive apneas. Neither type 3 nor type 4 portable monitors record electroencephalogram, eye movements, and electromyogram activity of the chin and anterior tibialis muscles. Therefore it is not possible to determine whether the patient is awake or asleep during the recording. Type 3 and 4 devices are not useful in diagnosing parasomnias such as nocturnal seizures, rapid eye movement (REM) sleep behavior disorder and periodic limb movement disorder.

The major advantage of type 3 and type 4 monitors is that the sensors can be self-applied by the patient at home, eliminating the need for a technologist to perform a home visit. Patients can pick up the monitor in the sleep laboratory and be instructed how to apply the sensors to themselves before bedtime and mail or bring the monitor back to the laboratory the next day. These instructions can be given in group sessions. An alternative approach has been to mail the monitor with an instructional video and brochure to the patient's home.

A major improvement in newer-generation monitors is their use of nasal pressure as a surrogate marker for airflow. Most validation studies to date that compared results of portable monitor testing with PSG have used older model portable monitors that used oronasal thermistors to measure airflow. Since those studies, nasal pressure measurement has become the preferred method for measuring airflow during sleep testing.[24–26] Oronasal thermistors detect only expiratory airflow, and their output is not linearly related to airflow. In contrast to thermistors, nasal pressure has a linear relationship with airflow over the range of tidal breathing, distinguishes inspiration from expiration, and reveals the presence of inspiratory flow limitation.

Although the classification of portable monitors is still in wide use, it is outdated. The technological advances achieved since that classification was created allow current portable monitors to be configured to perform type 2, 3, and 4 studies and record any combination of signals. In addition, advances in technology have resulted in new measurement techniques that are not considered by the current classification scheme. Another weakness of the current classification system is the lack of standardization of portable monitors. Even monitors within a particular class differ widely not only in the number and types of signals recorded but also in the sensors used to record the signals, and the electronic processing of the signals. The wide diversity in portable monitors complicates the ability to compare results across monitors and generalize results obtained with 1 particular monitor. As stated in a recent practice parameters statement on portable monitor testing, "There is no universally accepted platform for generating simplified studies in the diagnosis of OSA. This means that results obtained for a particular device are applicable to that device and cannot be extrapolated to other devices, even those of the same class."[27] This lack of uniformity limits the ability to perform meta-analyses and evidence-based reviews. Previous evidence-based reviews have evaluated the results of research studies performed using monitors within a particular category without consideration of the technological differences that exist among these monitors. To advance the field, further standardization of portable monitors is needed.

WHICH PORTABLE SLEEP MONITOR IS OPTIMAL?

The type of monitor that should be used to diagnose sleep apnea in an unattended setting is likely to depend on the patient population to which it is being applied. For example, in a patient population with a high prevalence of congestive heart failure, one might want to use a portable monitor capable of distinguishing central from obstructive apneas and revealing the waxing-waning respiratory pattern of Cheyne-Stokes breathing (Fig. 1). Such a monitor would need an airflow signal and a signal to detect the presence or absence of respiratory effort. In contrast, the need for a monitor with a respiratory effort signal would be less important in a patient population with a high risk for OSA. For example, in the 4-site Sleep AHEAD study, 304 obese adults (body mass index [BMI, calculated as weight in kilograms divided by the square of height in meters] 36.3 ± 5.6 kg/m^2, mean $\pm$ standard deviation) with type 2 diabetes performed home unattended polysomnograms with a type 2 monitor. Scoring the studies using the AASM

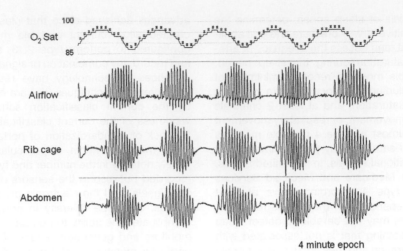

Fig. 1. A type 3 portable monitor recording showing central apneas and the waxing-waning pattern of Cheyne-Stokes respiration. A portable monitor that provides airflow and respiratory effort signals is capable of distinguishing patients with central sleep apnea/Cheyne-Stokes respiration from those with OSA. The sine wave pattern of the transient desaturation events is characteristic of this type of sleep apnea.

recommended criteria (hypopneas associated with at least a 4% oxygen desaturation), 87% of the patients had an AHI greater than 5 events/h. Only 1 patient had central sleep apnea (ie, >50% of the apneas were obstructive). All of the other individuals with sleep apnea had OSA. The high prevalence of OSA in obese patients with type 2 diabetes suggests that a type 4 monitor should be sufficient to diagnose their sleep apnea.

Pulse oximetry is widely used in type 4 monitors. Oximetry is appealing because of its widespread availability, reliability, and ease of application. However, the ability of pulse oximetry alone to detect sleep disordered breathing depends on the patient population selected for testing. Oxygen desaturation caused by a transient reduction in airflow is less likely to occur in nonobese patients without underlying lung disease. Individuals with an arterial Po_2 greater than 90 mm Hg at baseline are on the flat portion of the oxyhemoglobin desaturation curve and only minimal oxygen desaturation will occur even though oxygen tension during a period of shallow breathing decreases to 70 to 80 mm Hg (**Fig. 2**). The oxygen saturation signal in these patients is in the blind zone. Therefore, the use of pulse oximetry alone to detect OSA in the general population for OSA is likely to result in missed diagnoses (false-negative studies). In contrast, patients who are obese and have pulmonary parenchymal disease are more likely to have a reduced arterial Po_2 during wakefulness at rest that is closer to the inflection point of the oxyhemoglobin desaturation curve. A decrease in oxygen tension associated with shallow breathing therefore results in a relatively large decrease

in oxygen saturation. For example, in the obese patients with type 2 diabetes who participated in Sleep AHEAD, the mean AHI was 20.5 $\pm$ 16.8 events/h and the mean oxygen desaturation index was 17.6 $\pm$ 14.7 events/h.[28] The similarity of these 2 measures suggests that overnight pulse oximetry may be an adequate diagnostic test for OSA in obese, type 2 diabetics.

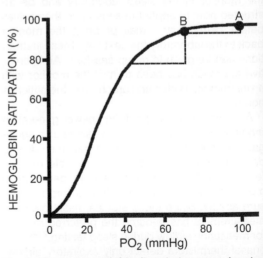

Fig. 2. The oxyhemoglobin dissociation curve showing hemoglobin saturation (Sao_2) at different arterial oxygen tensions (Pao_2). In a normal adult with a resting oxygen tension of about 90 mm Hg (A), a decrease in oxygen tension by about 20 mm Hg results in only a slight decrease in oxygen saturation. However, in a person whose resting Pao_2 is less than 80 mm Hg (B), a similar decrease in oxygen tension results in a larger decrease in oxygen saturation.

The type of monitor that should be used to diagnose sleep apnea in an unattended setting is also likely to depend on the resources and expertise of the health care facility performing the study. Some portable monitors provide automated scoring with or without the ability to perform manual review. Automated scoring is generally imprecise and prone to error. Manual scoring requires the effort of trained personnel. The AASM recommends that the portable monitor testing must allow review of the raw signals and manual scoring of the studies.[13] Portable monitor testing requires less technical expertise than PSG and is being used by providers outside sleep medicine, including dentists and cardiologists. However, lack of adequate sleep training may preclude their ability to accurately assess the results.

Another important consideration in selecting a portable monitor is whether its use is to diagnose patients with a high pretest likelihood of OSA or whether it should exclude as well as include the diagnosis. The answer to this question is related to the pretest likelihood of the patient population under study. In most current clinical settings, type 3 portable monitors are primarily used to test patients referred to sleep centers for evaluation of OSA. These patients have relatively high pretest likelihood for the diagnosis and most tests are likely to be positive. Using portable monitors in the general population to both include and exclude the diagnosis of OSA would likely increase the number of negative studies. Given the current technical limitations of type 3 and type 4 monitors,

it is recommended that symptomatic patients with a negative recording have in-laboratory PSG to exclude the possibility of a false-negative study for OSA and a non-OSA sleep disorder.[29] Use of portable monitors in the general population could conceivably increase the percentage of negative studies and increase the demand for in-laboratory PSG. Clinical prediction rules, including the Multivariable Apnea Prediction Index, Sleep Apnea Clinical Score, and Berlin Questionnaire, have been used to identify individuals with a high pretest likelihood of OSA in primary care practice settings. This strategy could reduce the number of false-negative results on portable monitor testing. However, use of these instruments has been confined to research studies and they have not been adequately tested in clinical management pathways.[30–33]

INTERPRETING TYPE 3 AND 4 PORTABLE MONITOR RECORDINGS

Despite the reduced number of signals recorded by type 3 and type 4 monitors, careful review of the raw signals may allow one to make inferences that can assist in interpreting the results. For example, note the transient increase in heart rate that occurs at the end of the apneic events in **Fig. 3**. This increase is likely because of the increase in sympathetic tone associated with an arousal. Therefore, although the recording does not allow arousals to be scored because of the absence of an EEG signal, these changes in heart

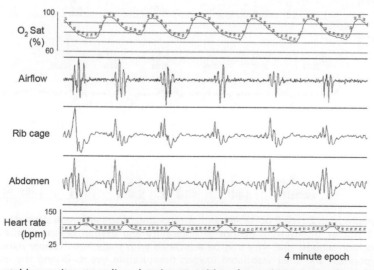

Fig. 3. A type 3 portable monitor recording showing repetitive obstructive apneas. The respiratory events are associated with marked oxygen desaturation that has the characteristic check-mark pattern seen in obstructive events (ie, a slow desaturation followed by rapid reoxygenation). In this example, the termination of the apneic episodes is associated with a transient increase in heart rate, probably secondary to an increase in sympathetic activity associated with an arousal.

rate, when present, provide indirect evidence that an arousal may have occurred at the termination of the event.

Although type 4 recordings are not recommended in patients with central sleep apnea/Cheyne-Stokes respiration, the shape of the oxygen desaturations on review of the oximetry signal may alert one to the possible presence of central sleep apnea/Cheyne-Stokes respiration and lead to referring the patient for in-laboratory testing. The oxygen desaturation signal in patients with OSA typically shows a slow decline and a relatively rapid return to baseline (see **Fig. 3**). In contrast, the oxygen desaturation in patients with central sleep apnea/Cheyne-Stokes respiration typically has more of a sine wave configuration, with a cycle of about 60 seconds (see **Fig. 1**).

The possible presence of stage REM can be suggested on type 3 and type 4 recordings by the pattern of occurrence of the apneas and hypopneas during the recording. For example, in the recording from a type 3 portable monitor shown in **Fig. 4** (upper panel), the respiratory events with associated oxygen desaturation occurred in distinct clusters scattered throughout the night in a distribution characteristic of REM sleep. The patient was in the supine position throughout the night, indicating that this finding was not caused by changes in body position. Another explanation for the presence of apneas and hypopneas in distinct clusters is that these were the times during the unattended recording that the patient was asleep. A morning diary completed by the patient can provide helpful information concerning the perceived quality of sleep during the recording, including the time to sleep onset and the number and duration of awakenings after sleep onset.

Another finding on type 3 and type 4 recordings with pulse oximetry that is suggestive of stage REM is the presence of several periods of continuous oxygen desaturation scattered throughout the night that are not related to position and cannot be explained by apneas and hypopneas (see **Fig. 4**, lower panel). This pattern of oxygen desaturation in stage REM occurs in patients with moderate to severe chronic obstructive pulmonary disease (COPD).

INNOVATIVE SIGNALS AND APPROACHES TO PORTABLE MONITOR TESTING

Novel technologies have been developed for portable monitors that are not used in standard PSG.[34] For example, actigraphy has been evaluated as a surrogate marker of sleep and wakefulness to improve the calculation of AHI.[35] However, the

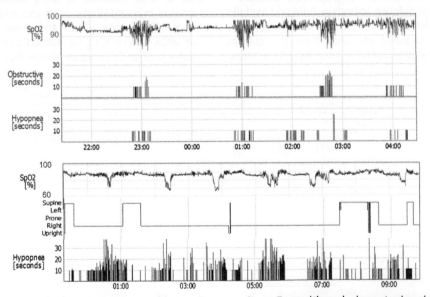

Fig. 4. Summary graphs from 2 type 3 portable monitor recordings. Even although sleep staging signals are not recorded in type 3 studies, intermittent periods of respiratory and oxygen desaturation events that are not related to body position suggest that they may be associated with stage REM. (*Upper panel*) The distribution of apneas and hypopneas and their associated oxygen desaturation events during the overnight recording suggest that the events were occurring in stage REM. The patient was in the supine position throughout the recording. (*Lower panel*) The 6 periods of continuous oxygen desaturation during the overnight recording are findings typically seen in stage REM in patients with COPD. These periods are not related to body position. Although this patient is having frequent hypopneas, they are associated with transient and less severe oxygen desaturation events that occur independent of the continuous oxygen desaturation periods.

restlessness during sleep that is characteristic of patients with moderate to severe OSA may result in the actigraph detecting movements during sleep that are interpreted as wake time, thereby underestimating sleep time and falsely increasing the AHI calculation. Another innovative approach is a type 3 monitor that incorporates the sensors that record nasal pressure, oximetry, head movement, snoring, and respiratory effort (venous pulsations) on a headband placed around the forehead.[36] Some monitors incorporate other novel sensors that detect cardiac and autonomic responses to sleep disordered breathing. One such device measures peripheral artery tone from a sensor on the finger that estimates changes in vascular flow, a measure that reflects variations in breathing and sleep-related arousals.[37,38] The technological advances in portable monitors outstrips our knowledge about their usefulness in clinical practice and it is possible that some of these unconventional signals may yield better diagnostic accuracy than the PSG respiratory-related measures recorded by most portable monitors.

VALIDATING PORTABLE MONITOR TESTING TO PSG

Initial studies to validate the use of portable monitors for the diagnosis of OSA compared the measures obtained on portable monitor testing with those obtained on in-laboratory PSG. Simultaneous portable monitor and PSG recordings can be obtained in-laboratory attended by a technologist and compared with portable monitor tests obtained in the home unattended setting. Differences in equipment and testing environments, and the known night-to-night variability in AHI, even on in-laboratory PSG, help explain why these direct comparisons have failed to find a close relationship between results from portable monitor testing and PSG. Type 3 and type 4 monitors do not record signals used to stage sleep and therefore cannot detect whether the patient is awake or asleep during the recording. The severity of the sleep disordered breathing on these recordings is quantified as the number of apneas and hypopneas per hour of recording, instead of per hour of sleep. The resulting measure is sometimes referred to as the respiratory disturbance index (RDI) rather than the AHI. Type 3 and type 4 monitors can underestimate the AHI that would have been obtained by PSG in patients with delayed sleep onset and low sleep efficiency. Although the relationship between in-laboratory PSG and type 3 and type 4 monitor testing is generally acceptable when the recordings are performed simultaneously in the sleep laboratory, the results

of studies comparing portable monitor recordings with PSG in the sleep laboratory may not be applicable to testing in the home setting (the intended location for portable monitor testing). Comparison across nights and in different environments results in greater differences between in-laboratory PSG and these home sleep studies. For example, patients are more likely to sleep in the supine position during in-laboratory PSG than during portable monitor testing at home, and any positional differences between the 2 tests must be taken into account in the data analysis.

VALIDATING PORTABLE MONITOR TESTING IN COMPARATIVE EFFECTIVENESS STUDIES

The recognized weakness of directly comparing portable monitor testing with PSG has led investigators to validate portable monitor testing by performing comparative effectiveness studies to evaluate clinical outcomes in patients randomized to ambulatory management pathways using portable monitor testing versus traditional in-laboratory PSG-based management. Patients randomized to each pathway are then initiated on positive airway pressure therapy and reassessed after weeks to months of treatment. Clinical outcomes in these trials have included improvement in symptom scores, self-reported quality of life, objectively measured adherence to continuous positive airway pressure (CPAP) treatment, and treatment efficacy (eg, AHI on in-laboratory PSG on the positive airway pressure used for treatment).

The ongoing VSATT (Veterans Sleep Apnea Treatment Trial), a 2-site study funded by Veterans Affairs Health Services Research & Development (S. Kuna and C. Atwood, principal investigators), provides an example of this study design (Fig. 5). In VSATT, participants randomized to in-laboratory testing were scheduled for overnight PSG in the sleep center.[39] If the AHI was greater then 20 events/h on the first 2 hours of sleep, the technologist was instructed to perform a manual CPAP titration in the remaining portion of the study (ie, split-night PSG). Subjects in whom split-night PSG established the diagnosis of OSA and determined an optimal CPAP setting were initiated on CPAP treatment. When full-night diagnostic PSG was performed, those subjects with an AHI of 15 or more events/h were scheduled for full-night manual CPAP titration PSG. Subjects who did not have OSA on PSG (ie, an AHI<5 events/h) were withdrawn from the study. Subjects with an AHI of 5 or more but less than 15 events/h on full-night diagnostic PSG were scheduled for a follow-up appointment in sleep clinic. During that clinic visit, if the sleep physician and patient

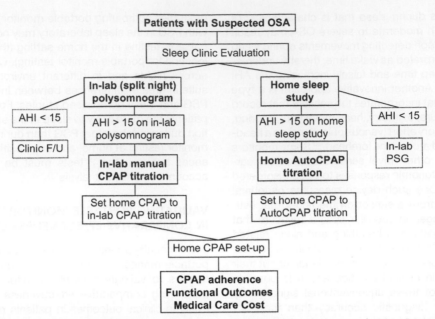

Fig. 5. In-laboratory PSG versus ambulatory clinical testing pathways for patients with OSA. Comparative effectiveness studies use this type of study design to evaluate whether the ambulatory management pathway differs from in-laboratory testing in terms of clinical outcomes such as CPAP adherence and daytime function. These randomized controlled trials can also compare the cost-effectiveness of ambulatory versus in-laboratory management.

decided that CPAP treatment was clinically indicated (eg, because of the presence of symptoms such as excessive daytime sleepiness), the patient was scheduled for in-laboratory manual CPAP titration PSG to initiate CPAP treatment.

Participants randomized to home testing performed a self-administered, overnight unattended sleep study at home with a type 3 portable monitor. Individuals with an AHI of 15 or more events/h on the home recording were scheduled for a 4-day to 5-day home unattended auto-CPAP titration study to determine the fixed pressure needed for CPAP treatment. Those subjects with an AHI of less than 15 events/h on the home diagnostic study were scheduled for in-laboratory PSG. Subjects in whom PSG could be split (ie, established the diagnosis of OSA and determined the fixed CPAP setting) were initiated on CPAP treatment. Otherwise, full-night diagnostic PSG was performed and those subjects with an AHI of 15 or more events/h were scheduled for a home auto-CPAP titration study. Participants with an AHI of less than 15 events/h on full-night diagnostic PSG were scheduled for a follow-up appointment in sleep clinic. During that clinic visit, if the sleep physician and patient decided to pursue CPAP treatment, the patient was scheduled for a home auto-CPAP titration study to initiate treatment.

Other ambulatory pathways need to be evaluated, including ones that use different AHI cutoffs

for decision making, compare different types of portable monitors, and evaluate treatment with auto-CPAP. However, any ambulatory management pathway must include the ability to perform in-laboratory testing on patients who are unable to perform home testing and patients whose results on home testing require them to be switched to an in-laboratory evaluation (eg, patients with central sleep apnea/Cheyne-Stokes respiration and symptomatic patients with a negative home sleep study).

USE OF AUTO-CPAP TO DETERMINE THE PRESSURE SETTING NEEDED FOR CPAP TREATMENT

The use of home unattended portable monitor testing to diagnose patients with OSA will be able to alleviate the growing demand for in-laboratory testing only if those patients diagnosed with OSA can be initiated on CPAP treatment without requiring PSG to establish the optimal CPAP setting. One alternative approach to in-laboratory CPAP titration by PSG has been to initiate CPAP treatment by selecting an arbitrary pressure based on measures such as BMI and instructing patients how to self-adjust the pressure setting at home.[40–43] A more common approach has been the use of auto-CPAP machines that automatically adjust the level of positive airway pressure delivered to the patient to eliminate their sleep disordered breathing.[44] The first-generation auto-CPAP models used a pressure adjustment algorithm based on the presence or absence of snoring and apneas and were often unsuccessful in adequately controlling the sleep disordered breathing. That problem has been corrected in newer-generation auto-CPAP models that include the presence or absence of flow limitation in inspiration, a more sensitive detector of airway narrowing, in their pressure adjustment algorithms. When pressure sensors in the machine detect the presence of snoring, apneas, or inspiratory flow limitation, the pressure in the circuit is increased. Absence of these feedback signals leads to a decrement in pressure. The algorithm for pressure adjustment is not standardized and varies across manufacturers.

OPTIMAL ROLE OF AUTO-CPAP MACHINES

No consensus exists regarding the optimal role of auto-CPAP machines in the clinical management of patients with OSA. Auto-CPAP has been used to titrate the fixed pressure setting needed for CPAP treatment in attended and unattended settings. It is also being used increasingly for long-term treatment of OSA. Unlike the in-laboratory manual CPAP titration polysomnogram that determines the fixed CPAP pressure in 1 night (or half a night) in a strange environment, an auto-CPAP titration can determine the optimal pressure setting by having a patient use an auto-CPAP apparatus for 1 or more nights in their own home. It is unknown how many nights auto-CPAP should be used during home unattended titration studies to obtain an optimal pressure setting. Auto-CPAP downloads report the daily pressure profiles delivered as well as the number of apneas and hypopneas, the AHI, and the amount of air leak from the mask. The downloads also report the amount of time spent at given pressures and respiratory parameters at those pressures. The fixed pressure selected for CPAP treatment is the pressure below which the patient spends 90% to 95% of the time. A significant drawback of the auto-CPAP downloads is the lack of published information validating the ability of auto-CPAPs to detect apneas and hypopneas, and therefore the accuracy of their estimated AHI determinations.

Auto-CPAPs are being used as regular treatment of some patients with OSA and seem to have particular usefulness in those patients who have difficulty tolerating high levels of CPAP throughout the night.[45] An arguable but untested approach might be to treat all patients with OSA with auto-CPAP instead of CPAP, obviating expensive in-laboratory CPAP titrations and eliminating

the concern that a fixed pressure determined on in-laboratory PSG (or home auto-CPAP titration) is adequate over long periods despite fluctuations in nasal airway resistance, body position, and body weight. Auto-CPAP machines are more expensive than CPAP machines, but, as the cost of auto-CPAP machines declines, this latter approach may become economically justifiable.

PATIENT SAFETY WITH AUTO-CPAP UNITS

To prevent adverse events related to excessive pressure delivery, auto-CPAP machines are limited to a pressure range from 4 to 20 cm H_2O or higher. Some patients with OSA can develop central apneas while receiving positive airway pressure treatment, so-called complex OSA, and further increases in pressure after the appearance of central apneas increases their occurrence.[46,47] Novel technology incorporated into the latest generation of auto-CPAP machines is able to distinguish if periods of airflow cessation are caused by central or obstructive apneas. When a period of airflow cessation is detected, the unit generates a short sequence of small, rapid pressure fluctuations. The resulting presence or absence of airflow in response to the pressure fluctuations allows the unit to determine if the airway is open or closed. The auto-CPAP machine increases the pressure setting when a closed airway is detected (ie, presence of upper airway obstruction), but does not increase the pressure setting if the airway is determined to be open (ie, a central apnea). A patient with an unattended auto-CPAP download showing persistent apneas should be scheduled for in-laboratory positive airway pressure titration PSG.

Some auto-CPAPs are designed to interface with other monitors to help ensure the adequacy of pressure titration. To document that auto-CPAP treatment is successful not only in controlling the apneas and hypopneas but also restoring oxygen saturation to acceptable levels, some auto-CPAPs can interface with pulse oximeter modules that record oxygen saturation and heart rate. Some auto-CPAPs are also designed to interface with a type 3 or type 4 portable monitor, recording respiratory-related parameters but not sleep staging signals, for a verifiable documentation of AHI as well as oxygen saturation. The latest innovations in auto-CPAP machines allow remote monitoring of their use and performance by either modem or wireless transmission of recorded data. Although no studies have investigated the use of this innovative technology, it is hoped that the ability to remotely track events during the home titration will lead to early interventions that can promote successful titration and initiation of CPAP treatment.

VALIDATION OF AUTO-CPAP TITRATION STUDIES

Validation of the home unattended auto-CPAP titration study faces similar challenges to those confronting validation of portable monitors for the diagnosis of OSA. Of particular concern to anyone who has interpreted manual CPAP titration polysomnograms is the short amount of time that the patient may be on the optimal pressure selected for CPAP treatment, often preventing verification of its adequacy in all sleep positions and sleep stages. The time available to identify an optimal pressure may be particularly limited in split-night PSG. Similar to the approach with portable monitors for the diagnosis of OSA, initial attempts to validate auto-CPAP titration studies directly compared the 90 to 95 percentile pressure setting with the optimal pressure determined on in-laboratory manual CPAP titration PSG. Differences in environment and equipment could explain why the 2 determinations did not have the same result. Although the night-to-night variability of the optimal pressure on in-laboratory manual CPAP titration PSG is unknown, it is likely that changes from 1 night to another also play a role in explaining discrepancies between the home auto-CPAP and in-laboratory PSG determinations.

Randomized control trials[48–51] and case-based studies[52–54] report that auto-CPAP is successful in selecting a fixed CPAP level that reduces the AHI to less than 10 events/h in 80% to 90% of OSA patients. The auto-CPAP trials in all but 2 of these studies[49,54] were attended by a technologist or nurse in the laboratory. Depending on the method of selecting the pressure from auto-CPAP and the manual CPAP titration protocol, the pressures from the 2 determinations were usually within 1 or 2 cm H_2O. One study suggested that using auto-CPAP rather than traditional CPAP titration to determine a fixed effective pressure for treatment decreased the percentage of patients declining continuation of CPAP treatment at 6 weeks.[49] Almost all previous studies with auto-CPAP have excluded patients with chronic heart failure and COPD. Future studies need to evaluate the performance of auto-CPAP in these special populations.

Recognizing the inherent design weakness of studies that directly compare optimal pressure obtained by auto-CPAP titration versus standard PSG, recent studies compared the 2 titration methods by evaluating the clinical outcomes after initiation of CPAP treatment in patients randomized to either home or in-laboratory testing.[43,49,55,56] Overall, the results report similar outcomes across titration methods. For example, the prospective study of Masa and colleagues[43] randomized 360 naive patients with OSA into 3 groups that received one of the following: standard CPAP titration PSG, unattended home auto-CPAP titration, or CPAP treatment based on a predicted formula with home self-adjustment based on the bed partner's reports. After 12 weeks of CPAP treatment on the determined pressure, an in-laboratory polysomnogram on CPAP was performed on all participants at their particular pressure setting. With CPAP treatment, the improvements in subjective daytime sleepiness (change in Epworth Sleepiness Scale score) and AHI were similar in the 3 groups. No differences were detected in the objective adherence to CPAP treatment or in the dropout rate of the 3 groups at the end of follow-up. The investigators concluded that home auto-CPAP titration and predicted formula titration with domiciliary adjustment can replace standard in-laboratory titration. In a similar study design, Cross and colleagues[57] found no significant differences in CPAP adherence or functional outcomes (Epworth, Functional Outcomes of Sleep Quality, and Short Form-36 scores) after 3 months of CPAP treatment in patients randomized to in-laboratory CPAP PSG versus home auto-CPAP titration.

COMPARATIVE EFFECTIVENESS STUDIES OF AMBULATORY PATHWAYS FOR EVALUATION OF OSA

Several studies now conclusively show that, at least in patients with a high probability of OSA, a completely ambulatory approach in terms of diagnosis and CPAP titration is feasible and has equivalent outcomes to in-laboratory management.[55,58–60] A study by Whitelaw and colleagues[60] compared the ability of physicians to predict which patients with suspected OSA would improve with treatment, as defined by an increase in the Sleep Apnea Quality of Life Index, based on information from standard PSG or oximeter-based home monitoring. These investigators found physicians' ability to predict treatment outcomes was poor, with correct prediction rates of only 63%, but there was no significant difference between PSG and home-monitoring group, suggesting that full PSG was not necessary for initiation of treatment in a select group.

Mulgrew and colleagues[55] performed a randomized controlled trial comparing an algorithm using a type 4 portable monitor and automatic positive airway pressure (APAP) titration with one using standard in-laboratory PSG in 68 patients with moderate to severe OSA. After 3 months of fixed CPAP treatment, no statistical differences between the 2 arms were found in AHI on end-of-study PSG performed on the fixed CPAP setting, change in the Epworth Sleepiness Scale score, or change in Sleep Apnea Quality of Life Index score, but CPAP adherence was greater in participants in the ambulatory arm ($P = .021$).

Using a similar approach, Berry and colleagues[59] randomized 106 veterans with a high likelihood of OSA to either home portable monitor testing for diagnosis followed by APAP titration for those participants with an RDI equal to or greater than 5 events per hour or to standard in-laboratory PSG for diagnosis and CPAP titration. After 6 weeks of CPAP treatment, these investigators found no statistical difference in total score on the Epworth Sleepiness Scale, global score on the Functional Outcome of Sleep Questionnaire, CPAP adherence, or patient satisfaction between the 2 groups.[59] These studies used comprehensive algorithms, incorporating both portable monitoring to diagnose and initiate treatment of their OSA patients. The protocols were conducted by highly trained and specialized staff, providing thorough education to all patients, with tertiary site backup. It is unclear what impact these factors may have had in determining the outcomes.

Antic and colleagues[58] compared a nurse-led model of care using oximetry and home APAP with physician-led care involving standard in-laboratory PSG for diagnosis and CPAP titration in a multicenter randomized controlled trial and, after 3 months of CPAP treatment, showed no significant differences between the 2 arms in change in the Epworth Sleepiness Scale score, quality of life indices, executive neurocognitive function, CPAP adherence, and total patient satisfaction. However, the nurses in the trial had worked in sleep for a mean of 8.3 years and spent approximately 50 more minutes with patients than the physician-led group.[58]

The two most recent randomized, controlled trials (HomePAP and VSATT) compared the effectiveness of ambulatory versus in-laboratory management of patients with OSA. Home-PAP is a multicenter study funded by the American Sleep Medicine Foundation (C. Rosen, PI). The protocols of both Home-PAP and VSATT are similar to that shown in **Fig. 5**. In VSATT, objective CPAP adherence and changes in functional outcomes after 3 months of CPAP treatment were equivalent in participants randomized to the ambulatory versus in-laboratory testing pathways.[61] Similar results have been found by the Home-PAP investigators (C. Rosen, personal communication, 2010).

OUTCOME MEASURES IN PORTABLE MONITOR VALIDATION STUDIES

For outcomes-based comparisons of attended in-laboratory PSG versus ambulatory management pathways, what are the critical outcome measures that should be measured? Performing in-laboratory PSG on the CPAP setting determined by the in-laboratory and home testing interventions once the patients have been initiated on CPAP treatment is probably the most direct approach to evaluate the efficacy of the resulting treatment.[55] However, differences between testing pathways may also change a patient's attitudes and perceptions about OSA and CPAP, altering their subsequent adherence to CPAP treatment. This effect on clinical outcomes can be evaluated by measuring objective CPAP adherence and self-efficacy.[62–65] Differences in these measures across testing pathways might arise because of the greater amount of time health care providers interact with patients during in-laboratory versus home testing.[66] The 1 or 2 overnight attended polysomnograms performed in a sleep center to evaluate patients with sleep apnea afford greater opportunities for education and immediate support, factors that have been shown to improve patient adherence to treatment.[67,68]

Functional outcomes after CPAP treatment are additional important measures for comparing the effectiveness of in-laboratory versus home testing. Examples of functional outcome measures include: the Psychomotor Vigilance Task for objective assessment of daytime sleepiness, the Epworth Sleepiness Scale for subjective assessment of daytime sleepiness, disease-specific quality-of-life questionnaires such as the Functional Outcomes of Sleep Questionnaire and the Calgary Sleep Apnea Quality of Life Index, and general quality-of-life questionnaires such as the Short Form-36 and Short Form-12.[69–76] There is almost no information on how much CPAP treatment is needed to improve functional outcomes and it is possible that similar improvements are obtained despite differences in CPAP adherence.[77] Other outcomes, such as systemic arterial blood pressure, that are related to the potential long-term consequences of sleep apnea might be selected for evaluation. It would be beneficial if researchers developed a consensus on a core set of outcomes that would be included in future studies of this nature to build the needed body of evidence that would lend itself to meta-analysis and evidence-based reviews.

COST-EFFECTIVENESS

Recently, several economic analyses of diagnosis and treatment of OSA have been reported.[78–82]

Three of the studies used decision analysis (ie, no direct observation of the competing therapeutic options being evaluated),[78,81,82] whereas 2 were based on data from randomized trials.[70,71] Chervin and colleagues[82] used decision analysis and reported that PSG is more costly and more effective than either home testing or empiric therapy. These investigators found that it has acceptable point estimates for the ratio of the cost per quality-adjusted life year gained compared with home testing (13,400) and empiric therapy (9200). Reuveni and colleagues[81] also used decision analysis, and reported that the combination of PSG and attended partial monitoring is the most cost-effective approach to sleep evaluation. Unlike several other studies,[19,83,84] these investigators also reported that unattended home sleep monitoring was the most expensive (because of the need for repeated sleep studies as a result of data loss and diagnostic disagreement). A similar conclusion was reached by Golpe and colleagues[85] in their intrasubject comparison of in-laboratory versus either unattended or attended home diagnostic testing. However, this cost-minimization study was probably underpowered and suffered from a 33% failure rate on unattended home testing, a value that is higher than that reported by other investigators and 4 times greater than the rate experienced in our own pilot studies.

There has been only 1 prospective study evaluating the cost-effectiveness of ambulatory management of OSA. Antic and colleagues[58] compared a nurse-practitioner–led ambulatory management pathway with physician-led management using in-laboratory testing.[58] These investigators found similar changes in Epworth Sleepiness Scale score in the 2 groups after 3 months of CPAP treatment but a decreased study-related cost per patient of $1000 Australian in the nurse-practitioner–led pathway. Additional prospective studies are needed, including ones that consider total medical care cost and use health usefulness and patient preference measures that allow comparison with other medical interventions. Such evidence will support decision analysis evaluations of ambulatory management of OSA. Published studies using decision analysis have had little impact because the inputs needed for a modeling analysis are uncertain.[81,82] Prospective randomized controlled trials on cost-effectiveness are needed to collect the evidence under naturalized, realistic conditions that can be used for a modeling analysis. These data can then be used to perform decision modeling that will help sleep specialists decide whether to use the more expedient home testing versus accepting delays in obtaining in-laboratory testing. Modeling

on these data can also determine the usefulness of home testing in patient populations with different prevalence of OSA and the economic impact of increasing access to care. One study addressed whether it is better to use home testing sooner or whether it is better to wait for in-laboratory testing and concluded that earlier diagnosis and treatment was cost-effective compared with waiting.[79]

SUMMARY

The need for alternative approaches to manage patients with OSA will continue to increase given the cost of PSG, the limited number of laboratory facilities, the increase in obesity in many countries, and the growing evidence that treatment of OSA improves functional and cardiovascular outcomes. What role will portable monitors assume and will this be based on a solid foundation of evidence or acceptance based on unavailable resources and familiarity of use? To answer these questions, we need to further standardize the sensors and signal processing used in portable monitors so study results can be compared across monitors. More prospective, high-quality clinical trials are needed to compare home versus in-laboratory testing in terms of treatment outcomes in diverse patient populations. Cost-effectiveness protocols should be routinely incorporated into these clinical trials to collect the data that will allow development of decision analysis models that are based on facts, not assumptions. Perhaps a rational first step is to target portable monitors to include but not exclude the diagnosis of OSA. Current portable monitor technology seems to be most applicable in patients identified as having a high likelihood of OSA using clinical prediction rules, patients undergoing preoperative evaluation for bariatric surgery, and obese adults with type 2 diabetes mellitus. Alternative approaches should also be made available to underserved and remote populations that do not have access to PSG testing. Creation of practice-based networks might be 1 method to collect the needed data in health care systems that offer traditional and alternative clinical pathways.[86] The rapid evolution and expansion of the discipline of sleep medicine into a multidisciplinary specialty is likely to increase the application of alternative testing methods. As physicians in family practice and otolaryngology join pulmonologists, psychiatrists, and neurologists to specialize in sleep medicine, the desire to test populations outside the sleep center will increase and it is hoped promote the research needed to systematically develop these alternative clinical pathways.

REFERENCES

1. Young T, Palta M, Dempsey J, et al. The occurrence of sleep-disordered breathing among middle-aged adults. N Engl J Med 1993;328:1230–5.
2. Young T, Evans LK, Finn L, et al. Estimation of the clinically diagnosed proportion of sleep apnea syndrome in middle-aged men and women. Sleep 1997;20:705–6.
3. Kapur V, Strohl KP, Redline S, et al. Underdiagnosis of sleep apnea syndrome in U.S. communities. Sleep Breath 2002;6:49–54.
4. Young T, Peppard PE, Gottlieb DJ. Epidemiology of obstructive sleep apnea; a population health perspective. Am J Respir Crit Care Med 2002;165:1217–39.
5. McNicholas WT, Bonsigore MR. Sleep apnoea as an independent risk factor for cardiovascular disease: current evidence, basic mechanisms and research priorities. Eur Respir J 2007;29(1):156–78.
6. George C. Reduction in motor vehicle collisions following treatment of sleep apnoea with nasal CPAP. Thorax 2001;56:508–12.
7. Jenkinson C, Davies RJ, Mullins R, et al. Comparison of therapeutic and subtherapeutic nasal continuous positive airway pressure for obstructive sleep apnoea: a randomised prospective parallel trial. Lancet 1999;353:2100–5.
8. Weaver TE, Chasens ER. Continuous positive airway pressure treatment for sleep apnea in older adults. Sleep Med Rev 2007;11:99–111.
9. Marin JM, Carrizo SJ, Vicente E, et al. Long-term cardiovascular outcomes in men with obstructive sleep apnoea-hypopnoea with or without treatment with continuous positive airway pressure: an observational study. Lancet 2005;365:1046–53.
10. Flemons WW, Douglas NJ, Kuna ST, et al. Access to diagnosis and treatment of patients with suspected sleep apnea. Am J Respir Crit Care Med 2004;169:668–72.
11. Pack AI. Sleep-disordered breathing–access is the issue. Am J Respir Crit Care Med 2004;169:666–7.
12. Collop NA, Shepard JW, Strollo PJ. Executive summary on the systematic review and practice parameters for portable monitoring in the investigation of suspected sleep apnea in adults: co-sponsored by the American Academy of Sleep Medicine, the American College of Chest Physicians, and the American Thoracic Society. Am J Respir Crit Care Med 2004;169:1160–3.
13. Collop NA, Anderson WM, Boehlecke B, et al. Clinical guidelines for the use of unattended portable monitors in the diagnosis of obstructive sleep apnea in adult patients. Portable Monitoring Task Force of the American Academy of Sleep Medicine. J Clin Sleep Med 2007;3(7):737–47.
14. Flemons WW, Littner MR, Rowley JA, et al. Home diagnosis of sleep apnea: a systematic review of the literature: an evidence review co-sponsored by the American Academy of Sleep Medicine, the American College of Chest Physicians, and the American Thoracic Society. Chest 2003;124:1543–79.
15. Ross SD, Sheinhait IA, Harrison KA, et al. Systematic review of the literature regarding the diagnosis of sleep apnea: evidence report/technology assessment No. 1. Rockville (MD): Agency for Health Care Policy and Research; 1999.
16. Kuna ST. Portable-monitor testing: an alternative strategy for managing patients with obstructive sleep apnea. Respir Care 2010;55(9):1196–215.
17. Sunwoo B, Kuna ST. Ambulatory management of patients with sleep apnea: is there a place for portable monitor testing? Clin Chest Med 2010;31(2):299–308.
18. Trikalinos TA, Ip S, Raman G, et al. Technology assessment. Home diagnosis of obstructive sleep apnea-hypopnea syndrome. Department of Health and Human Services, Agency for Healthcare Research and Quality; 2007. Available at: http://www.cms.hhs.gov/determinationprocess/downloads/id48TA.pdf. Accessed August 8, 2007.
19. Ferber R, Millman RP, Coppola M, et al. Portable recording in the assessment of obstructive sleep apnea: ASDA standards of practice. Sleep 1994;17:378–92.
20. Redline S, Tosteson T, Boucher MD, et al. Measurement of sleep-related breathing disturbances in epidemiological studies: assessment of the validity and reproducibility of a portable monitoring device. Chest 1991;100:1281–6.
21. Foster GD, Kuna ST, Sanders M, et al. Sleep apnea in obese adults with type 2 diabetes: baseline results from the Sleep AHEAD study. Sleep 2005;28:A205.
22. Redline S, Sanders MH, Lind BK, et al. Methods for obtaining and analyzing unattended polysomnography data for a multicenter study, Sleep Heart Health Research Group. Sleep 1998;21:759–67.
23. Goodwin JL, Kaemingk KL, Fregosi RF, et al. Clinical outcomes associated with sleep-disordered breathing in Caucasian and Hispanic children–the Tucson Children's Assessment of Sleep Study (TuCASA). Sleep 2003;26:587–91.
24. Norman RG, Ahmed MM, Walsleben JA, et al. Detection of respiratory events during NPSG: nasal cannula/pressure sensor versus thermistor. Sleep 1997;20(12):1175–84.
25. Thurnheer R, Xie X, Bloch KE. Accuracy of nasal cannula pressure recordings for assessment of ventilation during sleep. Am J Respir Crit Care Med 2001;164:1914–9.
26. Montserrat JM, Farré R, Ballester E, et al. Evaluation of nasal prongs for estimating nasal airflow. Am J Respir Crit Care Med 1997;155:211–5.
27. Chesson AL, Berry RB, Pack AI. Practice parameters for the use of portable monitor devices in the

investigation of suspected obstructive sleep apnea in adults. A joint project sponsored by the American Academy of Sleep Medicine, the American Thoracic Society, and the American College of Chest Physicians. Sleep 2003;26:907–13.

28. Foster GD, Sanders MH, Millman R, et al. Obstructive sleep apnea among obese patients with type 2 diabetes. Diabetes Care 2009;32(6):1017–9.

29. American Sleep Disorders Association Report. Practice parameters for the indications for polysomnography and related procedures. Sleep 1997;20:406–22.

30. Flemons WW, Whitelaw WA, Brant R, et al. Likelihood ratios for a sleep apnea clinical prediction rule. Am J Respir Crit Care Med 1994;150:1279–85.

31. Maislin G, Gurubhagavatula I, Hachadoorian R, et al. Operating characteristics of the multivariable apnea prediction index in non-clinic populations. Sleep 2003;26:A247.

32. Maislin G, Pack AI, Kribbs NB, et al. A survey screen for prediction of apnea. Sleep 1995;18:158–66.

33. Netzer NC, Stoohs RA, Netzer CM, et al. Using the Berlin questionnaire to identify patients at risk for the sleep apnea syndrome. Ann Intern Med 1999; 131:485–91.

34. Institute of Medicine Committee on Sleep Medicine and Research. Ensuring adequate diagnosis and treatment: access, capacity, and technology development. In: Colten HR, Altevogt BM, editors. Sleep disorders and sleep deprivation: an unmet public health problem. Washington, DC: The National Academies Press; 2006. p. 261–80.

35. Elbaz M, Roue GM, Lofaso F, et al. Utility of actigraphy in the diagnosis of obstructive sleep apnea. Sleep 2002;25:527–31.

36. Westbrook PR, Levendowski DJ, Cvetinovic M, et al. Description and validation of the apnea risk evaluation system: a novel method to diagnose sleep apnea-hypopnea in the home. Chest 2005;128: 2166–75.

37. Penzel T, Fricke R, Jerrentrup A, et al. Peripheral arterial tonometry for the diagnosis of obstructive sleep apnea. Biomed Tech (Berl) 2002;47(Suppl 1 Pt 1):315–7.

38. Pittman SD, Ayas NT, MacDonald M, et al. Using a wrist-worn device based on peripheral arterial tonometry to diagnose obstructive sleep apnea: in-laboratory and ambulatory validation. Sleep 2004; 27:923–33.

39. Kushida CA, Littner MR, Morgenthaler T, et al. Practice parameters for indications for polysomnography and related procedures: an update for 2005. Sleep 2005;28:499–521.

40. Coppola M, Lawee M. Management of obstructive sleep apnea syndrome in the home. The role of portable sleep apnea recording. Chest 1994;104:19–25.

41. Fitzpatrick M, Alloway C, Wakeford T, et al. Can patients with obstructive sleep apnea titrate their own continuous positive airway pressure? Am J Respir Crit Care Med 2003;167:716–22.

42. Hukins CA. Arbitrary-pressure continuous positive airway pressure for obstructive sleep apnea. Am J Respir Crit Care Med 2005;171:500–5.

43. Masa JF, Jimenez A, Duran J, et al. Alternative methods of titrating continuous positive airway pressure: a large multicenter study. Am J Respir Crit Care Med 2004;170(11):1218–24.

44. Berry RB, Parish JM, Hartse KM. The use of auto-titrating continuous positive airway pressure for treatment of adult obstructive sleep apnea. Sleep 2002;25:148–73.

45. Nolan GM, Doherty LS, McNicholas WT. Auto-adjusting versus fixed positive therapy in mild to moderate obstructive sleep apnoea. Sleep 2007;30:189–94.

46. Gilmartin GS, Daly RW, Thomas RJ. Recognition and management of complex sleep-disordered breathing. Curr Opin Pulm Med 2005;11:485–93.

47. Morgenthaler TI, Kagramanov V, Hanak V, et al. Complex sleep apnea syndrome: is it a unique clinical syndrome? Sleep 2006;29:1203–9.

48. Lloberes P, Ballester E, Montserral JM, et al. Comparison of manual and automatic CPAP titration in patients with sleep apnea/hypopnea syndrome. Am J Respir Crit Care Med 1996;154:1755–8.

49. Stradling JR, Barbour C, Pitson DJ, et al. Automatic nasal continuous positive pressure titration in the laboratory: patient outcomes. Thorax 1997;52:72–5.

50. Teschler H, Berthon-Jones M, Thompson AB, et al. Automated continuous positive airway pressure titration for obstructive sleep apnea syndrome. Am J Respir Crit Care Med 1996;154:734–40.

51. Teschler H, Farhat AA, Exner V, et al. AutoSet nasal CPAP titration: constancy of pressure, compliance and effectiveness at 8 month follow-up. Eur Respir J 1997;10:2073–8.

52. Berkani M, Lofaso F, Chouaid C, et al. CPAP titration by an auto-CPAP device based on snoring detection: a clinical trial and economic considerations. Eur Respir J 1998;12:759–63.

53. Gagnadoux F, Rakotonanhary D, Martins de Araujo MT, et al. Long-term efficacy of fixed CPAP recommended by Autoset for OSAS. Sleep 1999;22:1095–7.

54. Sériès F. Accuracy of unattended home CPAP titration in the treatment of obstructive sleep apnea. Am J Respir Crit Care Med 2000;162:94–7.

55. Mulgrew AT, Fox N, Ayas NT, et al. Diagnosis and initial management of obstructive sleep apnea without polysomnography: a randomized validation study. Ann Intern Med 2007;146:157–66.

56. West SD, Jones DR, Stradling JR. Comparison of three ways to determine and deliver pressure during nasal CPAP therapy for obstructive sleep apnea. Thorax 2006;61:226–31.

57. Cross MD, Vennelle M, Engleman HM, et al. Comparison of CPAP titration at home or the sleep

laboratory in the sleep apnoea hypopnoea syndrome. Sleep 2006;29:1451–5.

58. Antic NA, Buchan C, Esterman A, et al. A randomized controlled trial of nurse-led care for symptomatic moderate-severe obstructive sleep apnea. Am J Respir Crit Care Med 2009;179(6):501–8.

59. Berry RB, Hill G, Thompson L, et al. Portable monitoring and autotitration versus polysomnography for the diagnosis and treatment of sleep apnea. Sleep 2008;31(10):1423–31.

60. Whitelaw WA, Brant RF, Flemons WW. Clinical usefulness of home oximetry compared with polysomnography for assessment of sleep apnea. Am J Respir Crit Care Med 2005;171:188–93.

61. Kuna ST, Gurubhagavatula I, Maislin G, et al. Non-inferiority of functional outcome in ambulatory management of obstructive sleep apnea. Am J Respir Crit Care Med 2011;183:1238–44.

62. Kribbs NB, Pack AI, Kline LR, et al. Objective measurements of patterns of nasal CPAP use by patients with obstructive sleep apnea. Am J Respir Crit Care Med 1993;147:887–95.

63. Weaver TE, Kribbs NB, Pack AI, et al. Night-to-night variability in CPAP use over first three months of treatment. Sleep 1997;20:278–83.

64. Aloia MS, Arnedt JT, Stepnowsky C, et al. Predicting treatment adherence in obstructive sleep apnea using principles of behavior change. J Clin Sleep Med 2005;1:346–53.

65. Stepnowsky CJJ, Marler MR, Ancoli-Israel S. Determinants of nasal CPAP compliance. Sleep Med 2002; 3:239–47.

66. Kreiger J, Sforza E, Petiau C, et al. Simplified diagnostic procedure for obstructive sleep apnea syndrome: lower subsequent compliance with CPAP. Eur Respir J 1998;12:776–9.

67. Hoy CJ, Vennelle M, Kingshott RN, et al. Can intensive support improve continuous positive airway pressure use in patients with the sleep apnea/hypopnea syndrome? Am J Respir Crit Care Med 1999; 159:1096–100.

68. Jean Wiese H, Boethel C, Phillips B, et al. CPAP compliance: video education may help! Sleep Med 2005;6:171–4.

69. Dinges DF, Pack F, Williams K, et al. Cumulative sleepiness, mood disturbance, and psychomotor vigilance performance decrements during a week of sleep restricted to 4-5 hours per night. Sleep 1997;20(4):267–77.

70. Dinges DF, Powell J. Microcomputer analyses of performance on a portable, simple visual RT task during sustained operations. Behav Res Meth Instrum Comput 1985;17:652–5.

71. Johns MW. A new method for measuring daytime sleepiness: the Epworth sleepiness scale. Sleep 1991;14:540–5.

72. Johns MW. Sensitivity and specificity of the multiple sleep latency test (MSLT), the maintenance of wakefulness test and Epworth sleepiness scale: failure of the MSLT as a gold standard. J Sleep Res 2000;9: 5–11.

73. Weaver TE, Laizner AM, Evans LK, et al. An instrument to measure functional status outcomes for disorders of excessive sleepiness. Sleep 1997;20:835–43.

74. Flemons WW, Reimer MA. Development of a disease-specific health-related quality of life questionnaire for sleep apnea. Am J Respir Crit Care Med 1998;158:494–503.

75. Ware JE Jr, Snow KK, Kosinski M, et al. SF-36 health survey manual and interpretation guide. Boston: The Health Institute, New England Medical Center; 1993.

76. Luo X, George ML, Kakouras I, et al. Reliability, validity, and responsiveness of the Short Form 12-item survey (SF-12) in patients with back pain. Spine 2003;28:1739–45.

77. Weaver TE, Maislin G, Dinges DF, et al. Relationship between hours of CPAP use and achieving normal levels of sleepiness and daily functioning. Sleep 2007;30(6):711–9.

78. Mar J, Rueda JR, Duran-Cantolla J, et al. The cost-effectiveness of nCPAP treatment in patients with moderate-to-severe obstructive sleep apnoea. Eur Respir J 2003;21:515–22.

79. Pelletier-Fleury N, Meslier N, Gagnadoux F, et al. Economic arguments for the immediate management of moderate-to-severe obstructive sleep apnoea syndrome. Eur Respir J 2004;23:53–60.

80. Planès C, D'Ortho MP, Foucher A, et al. Efficacy and cost of home-initiated auto-nCPAP versus conventional nCPAP. Sleep 2003;26:156–60.

81. Reuveni H, Schweitzer E, Tarasiuk A. A cost-effectiveness analysis of alternative at-home or in-laboratory technologies for the diagnosis of obstructive sleep apnea syndrome. Med Decis Making 2001; 21:451–8.

82. Chervin RD, Murman DL, Malow BA, et al. Cost-utility of three approaches to the diagnosis of sleep apnea: polysomnography, home testing, and empirical therapy. Ann Intern Med 1999;130:496–505.

83. White D, Gibb T, Wall J, et al. Assessment of accuracy and analysis time of a novel device to monitor sleep and breathing in the home. Sleep 1995;18: 115–26.

84. Whittle AT, Finch SP, Mortimore IL, et al. Use of home sleep studies for diagnosis of the sleep apnoea/hypopnoea syndrome. Thorax 1997;52:1068–73.

85. Golpe R, Jimenez A, Carpizo R. Home sleep studies in the assessment of sleep apnea/hypopnea syndrome. Chest 2002;122:1156–61.

86. Westfall JM, Mold J, Fagnan L. Practice-based research–"Blue Highways" on the NIH roadmap. JAMA 2007;297:403–6.

Uses and Limitations of Portable Monitoring for Diagnosis and Management of Obstructive Sleep Apnea

Richard B. Berry, MD

KEYWORDS

- Breathing • Monitoring • Obstructive sleep apnea
- Polysomnography • Portable monitoring
- Home sleep testing

The proper management of obstructive sleep apnea (OSA), a common disorder associated with significant morbidity and mortality, requires accurate assessment. Polysomnography (PSG) is the standard test for diagnosis of suspected sleep-related breathing disorders and for positive airway pressure (PAP) titration to choose an effective level of PAP for treatment.[1–5] Attended PSG is costly and requires highly trained personnel for adequate study performance and interpretation. Access to PSG in a timely manner is limited or delayed in some locales and has prompted use of limited channel sleep monitoring for the diagnosis of OSA. Such testing is sometimes called portable monitoring (PM) or home sleep testing (HST). The tests are not always performed in the home and can be performed in the sleep center or hospital. In addition, testing often does not determine the amount of sleep (no electroencephalogram [EEG] recorded). Hence the terms HST or PM are not ideal but are used in much of the literature on this subject. For simplicity, limited channel sleep monitoring is termed PM in this article except when discussing Medicare coverage, where the term HST is used. Although PSG is the standard test to diagnose OSA in the United States, more limited studies are routinely used in other locales. For example, Flemons and colleagues[6] stated in 2004 that, in the United Kingdom, PSG comprised approximately 10% of all sleep studies, with around two-thirds of studies being oximetry alone and the remainder being limited channel studies. PM is commonly used in the Veterans Administration (VA) Health Care System where the demand exceeds the capacity to perform PSG. However, despite the widespread use of PM in many parts of the world, such testing has only recently been approved for reimbursement and qualification of patients for continuous positive airway pressure (CPAP) treatment in the United States.

TYPES OF PM

In a 1994 American Sleep Disorders Association (ASDA) review of portable sleep recording, Ferber and colleagues[7] proposed a classification of sleep testing that is still in use today (**Table 1**). The original classification used the terminology level I, II, III, and IV testing but more recent terminology[8] characterizes sleep monitoring as types 1, 2, 3, 4 or types I, II, III, IV (Medicare). Type 1 sleep testing is attended PSG in a facility. Type 2 testing (unattended or ambulatory PSG) records similar parameters as PSG, although often a reduced number of parameters are recorded. Both types 1 and 2 testing allow sleep staging and scoring of arousals.

Division of Pulmonary, Critical Care, and Sleep Medicine, University of Florida, Box 100225 HSC, Gainesville, FL 32610-0225, USA
E-mail address: berryrb@medicine.ufl.edu

Sleep Med Clin 6 (2011) 309–333
doi:10.1016/j.jsmc.2011.05.002
1556-407X/11/$ – see front matter © 2011 Elsevier Inc. All rights reserved.

Table 1
Classification of sleep testing

	Level I (Type I)	Level II (Type II)	Level III (Type III)	Level IV (Type IV)
	Attended PSG	Unattended PSG	Cardiorespiratory monitoring	Continuous single or dual bioparameter recording
Measures (channels)	Minimum of 7 channels including EEG, EOG, chin EMG, ECG, airflow, respiratory effort, oxygen saturation	Minimum of 7 channels including EEG, EOG, chin EMG, ECG, airflow, respiratory effort, oxygen saturation	Minimum of 4, including ventilation (at least 2 channels of respiratory movement or respiratory movement and airflow), heart rate or ECG, and oxygen saturation	Minimum of 1, including oxygen saturation, flow, or chest movement
Body position	Documented or objectively measured	Possible	Possible	No
Leg movement	EMG or motion sensor desirable but optional	Optional	Optional	No
Personnel interventions	Possible	No	No	No

In Ref.[7] the terminology of level I to IV was used but recent terminology is type I to IV.
    Data from Ferber R, Millman R, Coppola M, et al. Portable recording in the assessment of obstructive sleep apnea. ASDA standards of practice. Sleep 1994;17:378–92.

Type 2 studies have been used in the Sleep Heart Health Study, a large population-based study of the effect of sleep apnea on cardiovascular morbidity.[9,10] However, type 2 studies are rarely performed in nonresearch settings because of the required expertise and limited reimbursement (compared with type 1 studies). A type 3 study, also called **cardiorespiratory testing**, consists of a minimum of 4 measures with at least 2 channels of respiratory monitoring, oximetry, and electrocardiography (ECG) or heart rate. The 2 channels of respiratory monitoring are typically airflow and respiratory effort but could be 2 channels of respiratory effort (eg, chest and abdominal respiratory inductance plethysmography [RIP]). In most type 3 devices, the heart rate is derived from the oximetry data. An example of a type 3 study is shown in **Fig. 1**. Type 4 testing consists of a single or dual bioparameter recording, which most commonly consists of oximetry with or without airflow (often nasal pressure).

In 2008 Centers for Medicare and Medicaid Services (CMS) decision on the use of PM to qualify patients for CPAP reimbursement,[11] a slightly different classification of HST was used

(**Box 1**, **Table 2**). CMS defined type IV testing as a minimum of 3 recorded channels of information. The specific types of channels to be used for type IV monitoring were not specified in the original document. CMS also defined the respiratory disturbance index (RDI) as the number of apneas and hypopneas per hour of monitoring time, which differs from the commonly used definition of RDI as the number of apneas, hypopneas, and respiratory effort related arousals per hour of sleep. In a later publication (CAG-00,405N),[12] CMS stated that type IV studies record 3 channels, 1 of which is airflow. In transmittal 96, it was later stated that direct measurement of airflow was not necessary and other technology to determine an RDI would potentially be acceptable, but further details were left up to the discretion of the local providers (https://www.cms.gov/transmittals/downloads/R96NCD.pdf). However, Local Carrier Determinations (LCDs) often do define a type IV device as one measuring airflow and 2 other channels (LCD 29949, http://medicare.fcso.com). Oximetry is almost always recorded in type 4 studies. In the recent CMS memo concerning home sleep testing, a combination of peripheral arterial

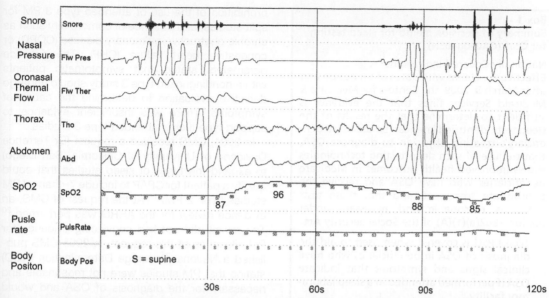

Snore	Snore
Nasal Pressure	Flw Pres
Oronasal Thermal Flow	Flw Ther
Thorax	Tho
Abdomen	Abd
SpO2	SpO2
Pusle rate	PulsRate
Body Positon	Body Pos

S = supine

30s   60s   90s   120s

Fig. 1. Tracings (120-second window) from a type (III) PM device (PDX, Philips Respironics) showing an obstructive apnea. Note the paradox in the thorax and abdomen tracings during the event. In this study, the signal from the oronasal device was suboptimal.

tonometry, actigraphy, and oximetry was accepted as a valid type of HST.[12] The older G procedure codes for portable monitoring (home sleep testing) and the new 2011 Healthcare Common Procedure Coding System (HCPCS) codes for portable monitoring are listed in **Box 2**. The new procedure definitions will likely require further clarification in the future.

TIME LINE FOR PM IN THE UNITED STATES

The history of PM in the United States is summarized in **Table 3**.[13,14] In 1994, an evidence review of the use of portable recording for sleep studies was performed by the ASDA (now the AASM).[7] A set of practice parameters for portable recording based on this review was published.[15] The 1994 practice parameters state that:

1. PSG is the accepted test for diagnosis and determination of the severity of OSA.
2. Unattended portable recording in the assessment of OSA is an acceptable alternative only in the following situations:
   a. Severe clinical symptoms indicate OSA and initiation of treatment is urgent and PSG is not readily available
   b. Patients are unable to be studied in the sleep laboratory (safety or immobility)
   c. As a follow-up study when the diagnosis of OSA was previously established by PSG and the intent of testing is to evaluate the response to therapy (weight loss, surgery, oral appliance).

The practice parameters recommended that body position be monitored and that a physician trained in sleep medicine and experienced in interpreting PSG should interpret PM studies.

In 1997, the Sleep Heart Health Study was launched using unattended PSG (type 2).[9,10] The same year, the practice parameter *Indications for PSG and Related Procedures* was published by the ASDA[1] **Attended** cardiorespiratory studies were said to be acceptable in patients with a high pretest probability of having OSA provided a PSG was performed when the cardiorespiratory study was negative in symptomatic patients. **Attended** cardiorespiratory studies were also acceptable for follow-up of non-PAP treatment of OSA to document effectiveness.[1] In 2000, a meta-analysis of evidence concerning diagnosis of OSA was performed by Metaworks for the Agency for Health Care Research and Quality (AHRQ).[16] The analysis did not find sufficient evidence to support use of portable monitoring for diagnosis of OSA. The wide diversity of device technology and study designs was a significant problem. Subsequently, a trisociety effort (American Thoracic Society, American College of Chest Physicians, AASM) was launched to review the evidence for portable monitoring. This initiative resulted in a systematic evidence review[8] and practice parameters[17] published in 2003 and an executive summary published in 2004.[18] The evidence review analyzed studies in which both PM and PSG were performed on all patients. The apnea plus hypopnea index (AHI) by PSG was considered the gold

Box 1
Summary of decision memo for sleep testing for OSA (CAG-00405N)

Nationally Covered Indications
Effective for claims with dates of service on and after March 3, 2009, the Centers for Medicare & Medicaid Services finds that the evidence is sufficient to determine that the results of the sleep tests identified later can be used by a beneficiary's treating physician to diagnose OSA, that the use of such sleep testing technologies shows improved health outcomes in Medicare beneficiaries who have OSA and receive the appropriate treatment, and that these tests are thus reasonable and necessary under section 1862(a)(1)(A) of the Social Security Act.

1. Type I PSG is covered when used to aid the diagnosis of OSA in beneficiaries who have clinical signs and symptoms that indicate OSA if performed attended in a sleep laboratory facility.
2. Type II or type III sleep testing devices are covered when used to aid the diagnosis of OSA in beneficiaries who have clinical signs and symptoms that indicate OSA if performed unattended in or out of a sleep laboratory facility or attended in a sleep laboratory facility.
3. Type IV sleep testing devices measuring 3 or more channels, 1 of which is airflow, are covered when used to aid the diagnosis of OSA in beneficiaries who have signs and symptoms that indicate OSA if performed unattended in or out of a sleep laboratory facility or attended in a sleep laboratory facility.
4. Sleep testing devices measuring 3 or more channels that include actigraphy, oximetry, and peripheral arterial tone are covered when used to aid the diagnosis of OSA in beneficiaries who have signs and symptoms that indicate OSA if performed unattended in or out of a sleep laboratory facility or attended in a sleep laboratory facility.

Data from Centers for Medicare and Medicaid Services M, 2009. Decision memo for sleep testing for obstructive sleep apnea (CAG-00,405N). Available at: http://www.cmshhsgov/mcd/viewdecisionmemoasp?id_227. Accessed March 3, 2009.

standard. The ability of PM to rule in and rule out OSA was determined. In many of the studies it was not possible to identify a single PM AHI cutoff value resulting in both acceptable sensitivity and specificity. From the evidence review, the practice parameters recommended only **attended** type 3 monitoring to rule in or rule out OSA and then with some qualifications.[17] The qualifications included a requirement for review of the raw data,

prohibition of the use of attended type 3 PM for split studies, and absence of comorbidity such as chronic obstructive pulmonary disease (COPD) or congestive heart failure (CHF). The practice parameters stated that symptomatic patients with a nondiagnostic type 3 study should undergo definitive evaluation to determine the cause of symptoms. There was insufficient evidence to support type II or unattended type 3 studies.

In 2004, CMS received a request (Dr Terrence Davidson of University of California, San Diego) to expand the types of sleep studies that could qualify a patient for CPAP to include 7-channel PM studies (type 2 PM).[19] At the request of CMS, an evidence review for the AHRQ was performed.[20] The review did not find convincing evidence for PM. Because of this request, in 2005 CMS published a National Coverage Determination (NCD) stating that PM studies were not reasonable and necessary for the diagnosis of OSA and would not qualify patients for CPAP.[21]

In 2005, an update of the practice parameters for the *Indications for Use of PSG and Related Procedures* was published by the AASM.[3] **Attended** cardiorespiratory studies were deemed acceptable in patients with a high pretest probability of having OSA. In 2007, CMS received a formal request from the American Academy of Otolaryngology-Head and Neck Surgery to reassess the NCD for diagnosis and treatment of OSA to include HST as an alternative to PSG.[22] After this request, the AHRQ commissioned 2 technology assessment reports: (1) home diagnosis of OSA-hypopnea syndrome,[23] and (2) OSA-hypopnea syndrome: modeling different diagnostic strategies.[24] The 2 assessments were performed by the Tufts-New England Medical Center Evidence-based Practice Center and were used to build the case that portable monitoring can be used effectively to adequately diagnose OSA and would not increase costs or timeliness to diagnosis. The first document[23] examined 95 studies that assessed the ability of sleep studies to predict response to CPAP treatment or usage in adults. It concluded that, because the AHI (or for that matter, other sleep study indices) does not accurately predict CPAP use, type 2 and 3 portable monitors are likely to work as well as PSG in selected populations for predicting a positive response to CPAP. The second document[24] examined mathematical models to simulate 6 different strategies for diagnosing OSA and treating with CPAP. The strategy using attended PSG in a facility followed by CPAP titration and treatment took much longer than strategies using PM. Various stakeholders presented evidence for or against the use of PM to the Medicare Evidence Development & Coverage Advisory

Table 2
Centers for Medicare and Medicaid Services (CMS) classification of sleep testing

Code	Type	Setting	Monitoring
	I	Attended in facility	Minimum of 7 channels including EEG, EOG, EMG, ECG/heart rate, and oxygen saturation
G0398	II	Unattended in or out of a sleep laboratory facility or attended in a sleep laboratory facility	Minimum of 7 channels including EEG, EOG, EMG, ECG/heart rate, and oxygen saturation
G0399	III	Unattended in or out of a sleep laboratory facility or attended in a sleep laboratory facility	Minimum of 4 channels and must recorded ventilation, oximetry, and ECG or heart rate
G0400	IV	Unattended in or out of a sleep laboratory facility or attended in a sleep laboratory facility	Minimum of 3 channels Direct measurement of airflow not required: transmittal 96 concerning the national carrier determination www.cms.gov/transmittals/downloads/R96NCD.pdf However, some Local Carrier Determinations require that one channel be airflow LCD L29949 http://medicare.fcso.com/Fee_lookup/LCDDisplay.asp?id=29,949&submitcode=Submit
——		Unattended in or out of a sleep laboratory facility or attended in a sleep laboratory facility	PAT, minimum of 3 channels including peripheral arterial tonometry, actigraphy, and oximetry

Abbreviation: PAT, peripheral arterial tonometry.
From Centers for Medicare and Medicaid Services M, 2009. Decision memo for sleep testing for obstructive sleep apnea (CAG-00405N). Available at: http://wwwcmshhsgov/mcd/viewdecisionmemoasp?id_227. Accessed March 3, 2009.

Committee (MEDCAC), an expert panel appointed by CMS. A concise summary of the process and testimony is provided in an editorial written by Dr Alejandro Chediak in 2008.[25] In 2007, the AASM published clinical guidelines for the use of unattended portable monitors in the diagnosis of OSA (Clinical guidelines for portable monitoring [CGPM]) in adults.[26] The guidelines provided a recommendation that PM be performed under the auspices of AASM-accredited sleep centers. A proposed CMS determination was published in 2007 to allow for public comment.[27] In 2008, a final NCD was published (240.4)[11] stating that unattended HST (types II, III, and IV) could be used to qualify a patient for CPAP reimbursement. Type IV HST was defined as 3 channels of recording. Patients are given 12 weeks to show adherence and benefit from CPAP treatment. The 2008 CMS decision did not address whether HST would be reimbursed. In 2009, a decision memo by CMS further specified that HST (types II, III, and IV) studies were reasonable and necessary for diagnosis of OSA (and therefore reimbursable) (see

Box 1).[12] In addition, a device using peripheral arterial tonometry (PAT), oximetry, and actigraphy was deemed an acceptable type of HST (PM).

Subsequently, LCDs by regional Durable Medical Equipment Medicare Administrative Contractors (DME MACs or DMACs) or private insurance providers were published, further defining requirements for the performance of HST (PM) (see Box 2). The initial health care common procedure system (HCPCS) codes for PM were temporary G codes G0398, G0399, and G0400 for types II, III, and IV HST, respectively. The current PM HCPS codes are 95800, 95801, and 95806 (see Box 2). The code 95800 includes devices determining sleep time as well as heart rate, oxygen saturation, and respiration (eg airflow or peripheral arterial tone). Devices formerly classified as type 4 fall under the 95801 code. Devices formerly classified as type III would fall under 95806. The reimbursement varies with region but is modest (see Box 2).

In 2011 the AASM published accreditation standards for Out of Center Sleep Testing (OCST).[28] OCST is the latest term used for PM (HST).

Box 2
Typical requirements for reimbursement for HST (PM) and reimbursement rates

- Treating physician who orders the study must perform a face-to-face evaluation. Evaluation must include:

  - Sleep history and symptoms including, but not limited to, snoring, daytime sleepiness, observed apneas, choking or gasping during sleep, morning headaches
  - Epworth sleepiness scale
  - Physical examination documents body mass index (BMI), neck circumference, and a focused cardiopulmonary and upper airway evaluation

- Sleep center performing HST study must be accredited by American Academy of Sleep Medicine (AASM) or Joint Commission (JCHO)
- Raw data must be reviewed by physician who is Diplomate of the American Board of Sleep Medicine (DABSM), Diplomate in Sleep Medicine by a member board of the American Board of Medical Specialties (ABMS), or an active physician staff of sleep center AASM or JCHO accredited
- G codes: note some Durable Medical Administrative Contractors (DMACs) still use G codes

  - G0398: HST, type II portable monitor; minimum 7 channels
  - G0399: HST, type III portable monitor; minimum 4 channels
  - G0400: HST, type IV portable monitor; minimum 3 channels

- 2011 HCPCS Codes for Portable Monitoring and Sample Reimbursement[a] (these vary by both DMAC provider and sometimes locality)
- **95800** Sleep study, unattended, simultaneous recording; heart rate, oxygen saturation, respiratory analysis (eg, by airflow or peripheral arterial tone), and sleep time

  - $202 Global
  - $144 Technical component
  - $58 Professional component

- **95801** Sleep study, unattended, simultaneous recording; minimum of heart rate, oxygen saturation, and respiratory analysis (eg, by airflow or peripheral arterial tone)

  - $96 Global
  - $44 Technical component
  - $55 Professional component

- **95806** Sleep study, simultaneous recording of ventilation, respiratory effort, ECG or heart rate, and oxygen saturation, unattended by a technologist

  - $182 Global
  - $117 Technical component
  - $63 Professional component

[a] Reimbursement is for Florida (not Miami or Ft Lauderdale) see http://www.trailblazerhealth.com/Tools/Fee%20Schedule/MedicareFeeSchedule.aspx.

AHI PSG VERSUS AHI PM

There are several potential reasons why the AHI by PM and PSG might differ (**Box 3**). The AHI by PSG divides the number of respiratory events by the total sleep time (TST) in hours. The AHI by PM divides the number of events by the hours of monitoring. The TST is always less than or equal to the monitoring time and is often shorter than monitoring time by an hour or more. Thus, even if the same number of apneas and hypopneas are detected by PSG and PM devices, the AHI will be greater by PSG because the TST is less than the total monitoring time. For example, if 100 events are recorded and the TST is 5 hours but monitoring

time is 6 hours, then the AHI by PSG is 20/h and the AHI by PM is 16/h.

The AHI values from PM and PSG studies may also differ if the respiratory sensors used in the studies are not the same; for example, using a thermal sensor to detect apnea and hypopnea during PSG and nasal pressure during PM.[29] If PSG and PM studies are on different nights, night-to-night variability may also contribute to differences in AHI. Many patients have a much higher AHI in the supine position or during REM sleep. In these patients, the relative amounts of supine and REM sleep contribute to night-to-night variability in the AHI. The effects of various amounts of supine and REM sleep on

Table 3
History of developments in portable monitoring

1994 PM Evidence Review	Sleep Monitoring: Levels I, II, III, IV Defined
1994 ASDA[a] Practice Parameter for Portable Monitoring	Unattended PM is an acceptable alternative to PSG in the following circumstances: 1. Patients with severe clinical symptoms of OSA and when initiation of treatment is urgent and PSG is not readily available 2. Patient unable to be studied in sleep laboratory (immobility or safety issues) 3. Diagnosis already established by PSG and treatment initiated and the purpose is to evaluate response to treatment
1997	ASDA Indications for PSG. Attended cardiorespiratory study acceptable in patients with high pretest probability of having OSA
2000	Metaworks analysis performed for AHRQ; systematic review of diagnosis of OSA finds insufficient evidence to recommend PM
2003 Trisociety Evaluation of PM (ACCP, ATS, AASM) Evidence review PM Practice Parameters	Attended type 3 studies may be used to rule in or rule out OSA provided certain limitations are met Type 2, type 4 studies were not recommended
2004 CMS receives request to reconsider use of PM studies and commission PM technology assessment 2005 CMS decision	AHRQ evidence review finds insufficient evidence to recommend unattended type II, III, IV PM CMS decision: PM not indicated for diagnosis of OSA

2005 AASM Practice Parameters for PSG and Related Procedures	Attended cardiorespiratory study (type 3) is an acceptable alternative to PSG
	• Diagnosis of OSA if:
	  ○ High pretest probability of OSA
	  ○ A negative type 3 study with patients with high pretest probability of OSA Is followed by a PSG
	• Before planned surgery for snoring or OSA
	• Following surgery for OSA: moderate to severe
	• To document effectiveness of an OA
	• After surgical or dental treatment of OSA and symptoms return

2007 CMS requested to revisit PM issue by American Academy of Otolaryngology-Head and Neck Surgery	Two AHRQ analyses were performed: 1. Technology assessment: home diagnosis of OSA-hypopnea syndrome 2. OSA-hypopnea syndrome: modeling different diagnostic strategies
2006–2007 AASM Portable Monitoring Task Force	Clinical Guidelines for Unattended Monitoring 2007 PM should monitor at a minimum airflow, respiratory effort, and oximetry PM should be performed under the auspices of an accredited sleep center
2008 CMS 240.4 Final decision	Unattended HST (Types II, III, IV) permitted to qualify a patient for CPAP
2009 CMS Decision Memo CAG-00,405N	HST types 1, 2, 3, 4, and PAT devices considered necessary and indicated to diagnose OSA and qualify a patient for CPAP and are reimbursable
2008–2010 Local Carrier Determinations and procedure codes for PM	Restrictions on who can perform HST fee schedule
2011 AASM published accreditation standards for Out of Center Sleep Testing (OCST)	http://www.aasmnet.org/resources/pdf/OCSTstandards.pdf

Abbreviations: AHRQ, Agency for Health Care Research and Quality; OA, oral appliance.
[a] American Sleep Disorders Association (ASDA), now the American Academy of Sleep Medicine (AASM).

Box 3
Reasons why PM and PSG AHI might differ

PM AHI<PSG AHI

- Monitoring time>TST (eg, 10/5<10/4)
- PM sensors dislodged during the night (decreased events recorded)
- Night-to-night variability in AHI
- Less supine time at home
- Less rapid eye movement (REM) sleep at home (uncommon)

PM AHI>PSG AHI

- Respiratory events scored when patient is awake
- Greater TST at home
- Ethanol intake at home?
- Night-to-night variability in AHI
  ○ More supine sleep at home (less common)
  ○ More REM sleep at home

PM and PSG AHI different

- Different respiratory sensors used with PSG and PM
- Different oximeter performance
- Variability in manual event scoring

---

the overall AHI in a patient with mild OSA are shown in **Table 4**. A study by Levandowski and colleagues[30] found greater night-to-night variability with PSG compared with PM (**Fig. 2**). Another study comparing PM and PSG found that patients had less supine sleep at home compared with the sleep center.[31] Having less supine sleep at home would often result in a lower PM AHI compared with a PSG AHI. In addition, if some events are missed by PM because of sensor

dislodgement for a portion of the night, this will also reduce the AHI. However, patients may sleep better at home and have a greater amount of REM sleep. Individuals may consume more alcohol at home. Some events might be scored from PM studies while the patient is awake. These factors would increase the AHI by PM relative to PSG.

Exact agreement between AHI values by PSG and PM is less important than correct classification of a patient as having OSA or not having OSA. Although AHI values of 30 and 50/h are different, both would clearly support a diagnosis of OSA. However, values of 3/h and 8/h are similar, but only 1 would support a diagnosis of OSA. PMs often have their greatest usefulness in patients likely to have a high AHI. Differences in AHI by PM and PSG usually have minimal impact on the diagnosis of OSA in patients with moderate to severe OSA who have a high AHI by either technique.

AGREEMENT BETWEEN PM AND PSG

The analysis of agreement between different diagnostic devices is complex.[32] The sensitivity of PM for detecting OSA using PSG as the gold standard is the number of positive PM studies times 100 divided by the number of positive PSG studies. The specificity is the number of negative PM studies times 100 divided by the number of negative PSG studies. A large number of false-negative studies reduces the sensitivity, whereas a large number of false-positive studies reduces the specificity of PM compared with PSG. The positive predictive value is the number of true positives by PM times 100 divided by the total number of

---

Table 4
Effect of proportions of supine and REM sleep on the AHI

	Supine NREM	Nonsupine NREM	Supine REM	Nonsupine REM	
Assumed AHI (no./h) in different conditions	5	2	30	10	—
Proportions of different conditions during 4 nights and the resulting AHI	Supine NREM (%TST)	Nonsupine NREM (%TST)	Supine REM (%TST)	Nonsupine REM (%TST)	Overall AHI (#/h)
Night 1	40	40	10	10	6.8
Night 2	30	65	0	5	3.3
Night 3	20	60	0	20	4.2
Night 4	70	10	20	0	9.7

Note: The AHI was highest on night 4 because the amount of supine REM sleep (as %TST) was the highest on that night.

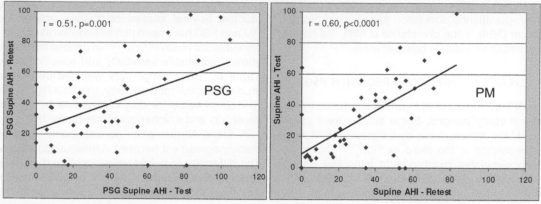

Fig. 2. The AHI in the supine position on nights 1 and 2 (test vs retest) in the sleep center with PSG are plotted on the left. The AHI in the supine position on nights 1 and 2 (test vs retest) at home with portable monitoring are plotted on the right. There was less difference between the 2 nights with PM compared with PSG. (*From* Levendowski D, Steward D, Woodson BT, et al. The impact of obstructive sleep apnea variability measured in-lab versus in-home on sample size calculations. Int Arch Med 2009;2:2; with permission.)

positive PM studies. For example, if the positive predictive value is 80%, then there is in the supine position an 80% chance that a positive PM study is correct. The positive predictive value depends on the prevalence of the disorder being diagnosed as well as the sensitivity and specificity of the diagnostic test.[32] The dependence of the positive and negative predictive values on prevalence is shown

in **Table 5**. Although the sensitivity and specificity are unchanged, the positive predicted value increases from 47.3% to 89% when the prevalence increases from 10% to 50%. At the same time, the negative predicted value decreases from 98.8% to 89.8% when the prevalence increases from 10% to 50%. Thus, a PM study with a given sensitivity and specificity will result

Table 5
Effects of prevalence of OSA on the positive and negative predictive value of PM compared with the standard test (PSG)

10% prevalence			PSG (the Standard)		
			Positive	Negative	Total
	PM	Positive	90	100	190
		Negative	10	800	810
		Total	100	900	
	Prevalence = (100/1000) × 100 = 10%				
	Sensitivity = (90/100) × 100 = 90%				
	Specificity = (800/900) × 100 = 89%				
	Positive predictive value = (90/190) × 100 = 47.3%				
	Negative predictive value = (800/810) × 100 = 98.8%				
50% prevalence			PSG (the Standard)		
			Positive	Negative	Total
	PM	Positive	450	55	505
		Negative	50	445	495
		Total	500	500	
	Prevalence = (500/1000) × 100 = 50%				
	Sensitivity (%) = (450/500) × 100 = 90%				
	Specificity = (445/500) ×100 = 89%				
	Positive predictive value = (450/505) × 100 = 89%				
	Negative predictive value = (445/495) × 100 = 89.8%				

Data from Flemons WW, Littner MR. Measuring agreement between diagnostic devices. Chest 2003;124:1535–42.

in a higher positive predictive value when used in a high-prevalence population (high pretest probability of OSA). If the prevalence is high, the negative predictive value is typically lower.

ACCURACY OF PM COMPARED WITH PSG

The AHI by PSG and PM can be compared using several study designs. Some studies have compared AHI values from simultaneous PSG and PM recording in the sleep center.[31,33] This approach eliminates night-to-night variability issues but is not the way PM devices are typically used. Other studies evaluating the accuracy of PM have compared the AHI by PSG in the sleep center with the AHI by PM at home (on a different night). A few studies recorded PM both simultaneously with PSG in the sleep center and at home on a different night.[31,33] In general, the AHI by PM and PSG tend to have better agreement when both record the same night of sleep (**Table 6**).

The trisociety systematic evidence review of PM for diagnosis of OSA analyzed a total of 51 studies published between 1990 and 2001. The studies analyzed included 35 type-4 monitors, 12 type-3 monitors, and 4 type-2 monitors.[8] Most of the studies excluded patients with comorbid sleep disorders or medical disorders such as heart failure. The PSG AHI results were considered the gold standard and the ability of PM to rule in or rule out OSA was determined. As noted earlier, finding a single PM AHI cutoff that was both sensitive and specific was problematic. The best evidence was for type-3 devices in the attended setting. However,

type-3 PM devices are rarely used for attended studies. Several studies comparing unattended PM and PSG have been published since the trisociety evidence review.[29–31,33,34] In general they have shown reasonable sensitivity and specificity (see **Table 6**). The findings vary with the population studied and the methodology. Use of a higher PM AHI cutoff value for diagnosis results in a lower sensitivity and a higher specificity for the test.

A Bland-Altman plot[35] is commonly used to display agreement between 2 measuring devices. The difference in paired values is plotted on the y axis and the average of the pair of values (device 1, device 2) is plotted on the x axis (**Fig. 3**). The mean difference between device measurements (bias) and limits of agreement (±1.96 times the standard deviation of the differences) are typically shown on Bland-Altman plots. Santos-Silva and colleagues[33] compared AHI values determined by a type III device (Stardust by Philips Respironics) at home with those determined by PSG as well as AHI values determined by simultaneous PSG and PM recording. A Bland-Altman plot of the AHIs determined with PSG in the sleep center with PM at home is illustrated in **Fig. 3**. Those points below zero signify AHI PM greater than PSG (overestimation of AHI by PM), and points above zero signify AHI PSG greater than PM (underestimation of AHI by PM). Two different comparisons between PSG and PM from the same study[33] are shown in **Table 6**. The first column is for comparison of AHI values by PSG and PM simultaneously recorded on the same night in the sleep center. The second column

Table 6 AHI by PSG and PM		
	PSG Versus PM (Simultaneous Recording in Sleep Center)	**PSG in Sleep Center Versus PM at Home**
Mean ± SD	AHI PSG 26 ± 28 AHI PM 27 ± 23	AHI PSG = 23 ± 24 AHI PM = 23 ± 24
Diagnostic agreement (%)	91	83
Overestimation of AHI (%)	8	10
Underestimation (%)	1	7
For AHI cutoff of 5/h		
Sensitivity (%)	98	93
Specificity (%)	62	59
Positive predictive value (%)	87	85
Negative predictive value (%)	93	76

Diagnostic agreement: AHI by PSG and PM both ≥30/h or AHI difference ± 10/h or less.
  Overestimation: PSG AHI less than 30/h, AHI PM > AHI PSG by 10/h or more.
  Underestimation: PSG AHI less than 30/h, AHI PM < AHI PSG by 10/h or more.
  Data from Santos-Silva R, Sartori DE, Truksinas V, et al. Validation of a portable monitoring system for the diagnosis of obstructive sleep apnea syndrome. Sleep 2009;32:629–36.

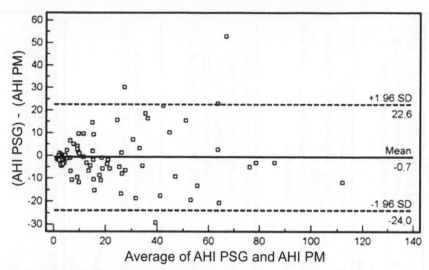

Fig. 3. A Bland-Altman plot of pairs of AHI values (device 1, device 2). The difference (device 1−device 2) is plotted on the y axis against the average on the x axis [(device 1 + device 2)/2]. The confidence limits are ± 1.96 standard deviation. The mean difference (bias) is near zero. There tended to be more scatter at the higher AHI values. (*From* Santos-Silva R, Sartori DE, Truksinas V, et al. Validation of a portable monitoring system for the diagnosis of obstructive sleep apnea syndrome. Sleep 2009;32:629–36; with permission.)

shows a comparison of AHI values between PSG in the sleep center and PM on another night at home. As expected, the diagnostic agreement is higher when recording is performed on the same night.

OUTCOME STUDIES USING PM

The ultimate decision of CMS[11] in 2008 to allow PM for diagnosis of OSA in patients to be treated with CPAP was heavily influenced by studies showing that clinical pathways using PM devices resulted in equivalent outcomes from CPAP treatment, including improvement in daytime sleepiness and the amount of adherence to treatment.[13,14,25] One of the AHRQ evidence reviews published in 2007 focused on outcomes rather than agreement in AHI.[23] Studies by Whitelaw and colleagues[36] and Mulgrew and colleagues[37] influenced the CMS decision (**Table 7**). Since those outcomes studies, others have been published showing similar findings.[38–40]

Whitelaw and colleagues[36] randomized 288 patients referred by a family physician to either standard PSG or a SnoreSat home monitor (only oximetry data were used). A randomly selected subset of eligible patients referred to the sleep center was studied. Inclusion criteria included a history suggesting OSA in association with somnolence or fatigue. Exclusions included significant comorbidity, absence of daytime symptoms, and significant physiologic consequences of OSA. Only 44% of patients were considered eligible

and, of those eligible, only 11% completed the trial. All patients underwent treatment with an autotitrating CPAP (APAP). The patients were followed after a 4-week period to determine their improvement with treatment. There was no difference in the ability of the AHI by PSG and the RDI by PM (desaturations/h) to predict the response to APAP treatment in terms of the adherence to treatment or improvement in the quality of life.

Mulgrew and colleagues[37] compared a pathway using PSG (diagnosis [Dx] PSG, CPAP PSG separate nights) with a pathway using autotitration followed by CPAP treatment (95% pressure). CPAP was further adjusted based on oximetry in this group. Patients were chosen based on the Epworth Sleepiness Scale (ESS), Sleep Apnea Clinical Score (SACS), and desaturations/h greater than 15/h. Thus, patients in both treatment pathways had a high probability of having moderate to severe OSA. Once patients met inclusion and exclusion criteria, they were randomized to the PSG pathway or the APAP pathway (oximetry→ autotitration→CPAP). At 3 months, the improvement in ESS and quality of life were similar between the 2 pathways. CPAP adherence was better with the pathway not using PSG (eg, oximetry→autotitration→CPAP). At the end of the study, PSG was performed on CPAP at the final pressure chosen for each patient. The 2 pathways had similar AHI values (similar treatment effectiveness). Only 81 of more than 2200 patients referred to the sleep center entered the trial. Exclusions included lack of subjective sleepiness, psychiatric

Table 7
Studies of clinical pathways using PM (outcome studies)

First Author	Patient Selection	Clinical Pathways	Outcomes
Whitelaw et al,[36] 2005	History suggesting OSA + symptoms of sleepiness or fatigue	Pathway 1: Oximetry for Dx (RDI) then treatment with APAP for 4 weeks Pathway 2: PSG for Dx (AHI) then treatment with APAP for 4 weeks	RDI and AHI had equal ability to predict improvement in quality of life and PAP adherence
Mulgrew et al,[37] 2007	High pretest probability ESS, SACS, then RDI >15/h based on oximetry (RDI = desaturations/h of monitoring)	Pathway 1: Dx PSG, CPAP PSG on second night, CPAP treatment Pathway 2: Oximetry for Dx, AutoCPAP titration, CPAP based on 95th percentile pressure and oximetry on CPAP to adjust pressure	Both pathways similar decrease in ESS and improvement in quality of life Higher median CPAP adherence with Pathway 2
Berry et al,[38] 2008	High likelihood of OSA and sleepiness (ESS ≥12)	Pathway 1: PSG for Dx and CPAP titration (most SN) followed by CPAP treatment Pathway 2: PM for diagnosis, autotitration for 3 nights at home, and CPAP treatment based on autotitration	At 6 weeks of CPAP treatment, pathways 1 and 2 resulted in equivalent improvement in subjective sleepiness, quality of life, and CPAP adherence
Antic et al,[39] 2009	Oximetry >27/h 2% or greater desaturations	Symptoms and oximetry for identification of high-risk patients/Dx then randomized to one of 2 pathways Pathway 1: Dx PSG, CPAP PSG, CPAP Rx Pathway 2: APAP titration, CPAP Rx	At 3 mo: No difference CPAP adherence No difference in improvement in ESS
Skromo et al,[40] 2010	Inclusion criteria: daytime sleepiness with ESS >10, witnessed apneas or snoring Exclusions prior CPAP or upper airway surgery.	Pathway 1: PSG for Dx and titration (most SN) then CPAP Rx for 4 weeks Pathway 2: (HM pathway) PM for Dx, APAP for 1 week at home then CPAP based on APAP	After 4 weeks of PAP treatment, equivalent CPAP adherence, improvement in quality of life, and ESS

Abbreviations: APAP, auto-titrating, auto-adjusting PAP; ESS, Epworth sleepiness scale; RDI, events/hour of monitoring time; Rx, treatment; SN, split night PSG.

disease, prior PAP treatment, low probability of having OSA, and unwillingness to use CPAP.

Berry and coworkers[38] compared a pathway using PM, APAP titration, and CPAP treatment with a pathway using PSG for diagnosis followed by titration (most PSGs were split studies) and CPAP treatment. Patients were required to have daytime sleepiness and a moderate to high probability of OSA based on history. An AHI greater than 5/h was used to diagnose OSA (by either PM or PSG) and all patients diagnosed with OSA were offered CPAP. After 6 weeks of CPAP treatment, the percentage of patients using CPAP, the mean CPAP adherence, and the improvements in ESS and quality of life did not differ between the clinical pathways. The study used a PM device based on PAT. This study was performed at a VA Hospital and more than 90% of the PM studies were positive for OSA.

Antic and coworkers[39] identified a high-risk patient group for OSA with ESS greater than 8 and oxygen desaturation index (2% dips) greater than or equal to 27/h. Patients were randomized to a pathway using autotitration, CPAP at the 95th percentile pressure, and treatment directed by specialist nurse (visits at 1 and 3 months) or a pathway consisting of diagnostic PSG, CPAP PSG, CPAP treatment, nurse visits, and MD visits if needed. At 3 months, the groups did not differ in ESS improvement or CPAP adherence. Of 882 patients who consented to be part of the trial, 263 were excluded based on clinical criteria. After screening with oximetry, only 195 patients met criteria for high probability of moderate to severe OSA and were randomized to the 2 study arms.

Skomro and coworkers[40] randomized patients to a PSG arm or home monitoring (HM) arm. In the PSG arm patients had an in lab PSG for diagnosis and CPAP titration (most split nights) and then CPAP treatment for 4 weeks. In the HM arm patients had a PM study at home (Embletta, Embla, Denver, CO, USA), auto CPAP for 1 week at home, and CPAP treatment for 3 weeks based on the autoCPAP results. Before the auto CPAP patients had a PSG titration that allowed comparison of the optimal pressure determined by PSG with the one determined by autoCPAP home titration. The pathways resulted in equivalent in CPAP adherence, improvement in ESS, and quality of life. The studies mentioned earlier suggest that diagnosis by oximetry or PM in a group with moderate to high probability of having OSA followed by CPAP treatment based on APAP titration results in equivalent outcomes compared with pathways using PSG. In all of the studies, patients with significant comorbidities were excluded. In some studies, a large fraction of the eligible patients did not enter the study. Thus, the study groups were often highly selected and evaluated by a team experienced in sleep medicine. The good results using PM pathways may not generalize to situations in which patients are not systematically evaluated before PM is performed and less experienced providers direct the PAP treatment.

CLINICAL USE OF PM
Advantages and Limitations of Type 3 (III) PM

There are several potential advantages of PM (**Box 4**), including sleep in the normal home environment with fewer sensors (patients may sleep better) and ease of study for patients with immobility, those with special needs (claustrophobia), or unstable medical conditions requiring intensive care. PM monitoring is less complex and less expertise is needed to set up PM and score the studies. The individual PM devices are less expensive than PSG devices. The number of diagnostic studies is not limited by the number of rooms in the sleep center. In locales with limited PSG capacity, use of PM may reduce the wait time to study and treatment. However, there has been a dramatic increase in the number of sleep centers[25] so access to PSG may not be limited in many locales.

PM also has several disadvantages. Some patients are anxious about becoming disconnected and would prefer an attended study. If sensors are dislodged during an unattended study, no technologist is available to intervene. A significant proportion of PM studies are technically inadequate (5%–30%).[41] PM testing is less cost-effective if a high proportion of studies must be repeated. PM devices are less expensive than PSG equipment but may not be returned or can be damaged in patient's homes. Type 3 or 4 PM studies do not determine the amount of sleep or amount of REM sleep. It may be difficult to determine whether a study underestimates the severity of OSA because of limited amount of sleep or REM sleep. Good-quality PM studies often require significant expertise in educating patients or hooking them up in the sleep center. Although PM studies are not as complex as PSG, they do require experienced personnel to avoid a high percentage of technically inadequate studies. Golpe and colleagues[41] found much higher rates of failed studies when the patients set up PM in the home (33%) versus having PM devices applied in the sleep center (7%). If the PM study is negative and the patient is sleepy, most patients will need a PSG. If the PM study is positive, many patients will need a PSG CPAP titration unless an alternative approach is available (APAP titration or

---

Box 4
Potential advantages and limitations for unattended type 3 PM

Advantages

- Sleep in normal home environment (patients may sleep better)
- Some patients may find PM more comfortable than PSG (fewer monitoring leads)
- Good for patients who are immobile or who might find PSG challenging (claustrophobia)
- Flexible setting: home, hospital room, hotel
- PM monitoring less technically complex than PSG
- Each device less costly than PSG equipment
- Less expertise need to set up PM device and sensors
- Less expertise needed to score and interpret PM studies than PSG
- Virtual sleep center: number of patients that can be studied is not limited by the size of sleep center
- In some locales there may be decreased wait times for diagnosis and treatment (depends on availability of PSG)

Limitations

- Some patients anxious about becoming disconnected without someone available for reconnection
- Unattended, so potential for monitoring leads becoming unhooked or technically inadequate study
- 10% to 15% technically inadequate studies (up 30% in some studies if patient places the sensors)
- TST and amounts of different sleep stages are not documented (type III and IV PM). Was TST and REM adequate?
- AHI underestimated because of division by monitoring time, which is greater than total sleep time
- May not determine amount of supine monitoring time (some PM devices)
- PM device loss or damage can be a significant problem
- Good-quality PM studies require trained personnel and have substantial costs (education, setup, download, cleaning units, analysis, report generation)
- Less cost to perform PM but much less reimbursement
- Need to perform PSG for negative studies in most sleepy patients
- If diagnosis of significant OSA is made, still need to perform PSG CPAP titration in most patients unless alternative approach used (APAP titration, APAP treatment, empiric CPAP level)
- Cannot detect arrhythmias if pulse rate by oximetry rather than ECG recorded

---

APAP treatment). A split study might be more cost-effective than diagnosis by PM followed by a PSG titration. The relative cost of the 2 approaches depends on the number of negative PM studies, the number of PM studies that need repeating, and the treatment algorithm once a diagnosis of OSA is made. In the private sector in the United States, autotitration studies are not reimbursed and durable medical equipment suppliers receive the same reimbursement for CPAP and APAP devices even though APAP devices are more expensive. These reimbursement issues limit the use of alternative approaches to CPAP titration and treatment.

CLINICAL GUIDELINES FOR THE USE OF PM
Attended Type 3 (III) Studies

The 1997[1,2] and 2005 updates[3] for indications for PSG stated that **attended** type 3 (cardiorespiratory) studies were acceptable for patients with a high pretest probability of having OSA, provided repeat testing with PSG is permitted in

---

Box 5
Indications for attended type III cardiorespiratory studies (airflow and effort [or 2 effort channels], oxygen saturation, and pulse or ECG)

- Diagnosis of OSA when PSG is difficult
  - Immobility
  - Safety issues
  - Clinical urgency and access to PSG is delayed
- Before surgery for planned upper airway surgery for snoring or OSA
- Postoperative after upper airway surgery for moderate to severe OSA
- Before oral appliance (OA) treatment of snoring or OSA
- After adequate adjustment of OA for treatment of OSA (all severities)

Data from Kushida CA, Littner MR, Morgenthaler T, et al. Practice parameters for the indications for polysomnography and related procedures: an update for 2005. Sleep 2005;28:499–521.

symptomatic patients with a negative type 3 study (**Box 5**). The 2005 update for practice parameters for PSG[1,3] also stated that PSG or an **attended** type 3 (cardiorespiratory) study was indicated for preoperative evaluation for planned upper airway surgery for snoring or OSA or for postoperative study after surgery in patients with moderate to severe OSA to document therapeutic effectiveness, or if symptoms return despite an initial response to treatment. The practice parameters for PSG also stated that attended type 3 PM was indicated for follow-up to document a response to an oral appliance in patients with moderate to severe OSA.[3] The practice parameters for the use of oral appliances (2005 update)[42] expanded the previous recommendations to include attended PM monitoring (with the oral appliance in place) for patients with all severities of OSA (mild, moderate, and severe). These recommendations have minimal relevance to clinical practice because PM studies are rarely performed as attended studies.

Unattended Type 3 (III) PM Studies

The 1997 practice parameters for portable recording[1] stated that unattended portable recording in the assessment of OSA is an acceptable alternative only when (1) severe clinical symptoms indicate OSA and initiation of treatment is urgent and PSG is not readily available, (2) patients are unable to be studied in the sleep laboratory (safety or immobility), (3) as a follow-up study when the diagnosis previously established by PSG and the intent of testing is to evaluate response to therapy (weight loss, surgery, oral appliance).

CGPM were published by the AASM in 2007 based on an evidence review and consensus.[26] The guidelines state that PM may be used as an alternative to PSG for the diagnosis of OSA in patients with a high pretest probability of moderate to severe OSA (provided certain conditions are met); in cases where PSG is not possible by virtue of immobility, safety, or critical illness; or to monitor the response to non-CPAP treatments for OSA (including oral appliances, upper airway surgery, and weight loss). In contrast with previous practice parameters, the CGPM state that **unattended** PM may be indicated for diagnosis of OSA in patients with a high pretest probability of having OSA if guidelines for patient selection and procedures for PM performance and interpretation are followed (**Box 6**).[26] PM is not indicated for screening asymptomatic populations. The CGPM also outlined recommendations concerning

---

Box 6
Indications and conditions for use of unattended PM (type III)[a]

Indications:

- Diagnosis of OSA in patients with high probability of having the disorder (without comorbidities or other sleep disorders)
- Diagnosis of OSA in patients in whom laboratory PSG is not possible by virtue of immobility, safety, or critical illness
- To document the efficacy of non-PAP treatments for OSA (oral appliances, upper airway surgery, weight loss)

Conditions:

- PM must be performed in conjunction with a comprehensive sleep evaluation supervised by a BC/BE sleep physician
- No comorbid medical conditions that may degrade PM accuracy

  ○ Severe pulmonary disease
  ○ Neuromuscular disease
  ○ CHF

- No clinical suspicion of other sleep disorders

  ○ Central sleep apnea (CSA)
  ○ Narcolepsy
  ○ Periodic limb movement disorder (PLMD)
  ○ Parasomnias
  ○ Circadian rhythm sleep disorders

- Not for screening asymptomatic populations
- Unattended PM in patient's home is acceptable[a] when all guidelines are followed

[a] The guidelines' wording stated that PM "may" be indicated.

From Collop NA, Anderson WM, Boehlecke B, et al. Clinical guidelines for the use of unattended portable monitors in the diagnosis of obstructive sleep apnea in adult patients. Portable Monitoring Task Force of the American Academy of Sleep Medicine. J Clin Sleep Med 2007;3:737–47; with permission.

---

technical aspects of PM and study interpretation (discussed below).

Patient Selection for PM

The CGPM state that a comprehensive sleep evaluation must precede PM. Ideally, each patient should be seen by a board-certified/board-eligible sleep physician before PM testing. If this is not possible, an evaluation can be performed with questionnaires or interview by a physician extender. The evaluation should occur before PM monitoring but, if this is not possible, clinical evaluation can occur at the time of testing.

> **Box 7**
> **Characteristics of good and poor candidates for PM**
>
> *Good*
>
> - High probability of moderate to severe OSA
> - No comorbid sleep disorders requiring PSG
> - No comorbid medical disorders degrading PM accuracy
> - Safety issues (need intensive care unit setting)
> - Immobility issues
> - Claustrophobia/unable to sleep in sleep center
> - Delay in PSG (long wait time)
>
> *Poor*
>
> - Low probability of OSA
> - High probability of need for attended PAP titration (split study may be more cost-effective than PM followed by PSG titration)
> - Comorbid sleep disorders
> - Comorbid medical conditions (making diagnosis by PM difficult or likely to require PSG titration)
>
>   ○ Moderate to severe COPD
>   ○ Hypoventilation, potent narcotics
>   ○ Low baseline Sao_2 or using supplemental oxygen
>   ○ High BMI, obesity hypoventilation syndrome suspected
>   ○ Moderate to severe CHF
>   ○ Nocturnal arrhythmias are suspected

Characteristics of patients who are good candidates for PM are listed in **Box 7**. Review of the medical record to exclude patients with comorbidities that may degrade PM accuracy is also important. In the CGPM, comorbidities excluding patients from PM include severe pulmonary disease, neuromuscular disease, or CHF. The rationale is that such patients may exhibit hypoventilation without discrete respiratory events or Cheyne-Stokes breathing (CHF). However, it could be argued that, if PM devices use the same sensors as PSG (the CGPM recommendation), then PM and PSG should have similar ability to detect central apnea, Cheyne-Stokes breathing (**Fig. 4**), or hypoventilation (manifested by a low arterial oxygen concentration [Sao_2] without discrete events).

According to the AASM scoring manual[43] a diagnosis of hypoventilation should be based on measurement of arterial PCO_2 or an accurate surrogate. Hence, neither routine PSG nor PM can definitively document hypoventilation. Although not specifically addressed in the CGPM, physicians should be aware that patients taking potent narcotics often have central apnea at baseline or with the application of PAP. Even if PM can detect

Cheyne-Stokes breathing, central apneas not of the Cheyne-Stokes type, or arterial oxygen desaturation without discrete events, patients with these findings would not be good candidates for autotitration or treatment with an autotitrating device. These patients will likely benefit from a PSG titration. Patients with a low baseline Sao_2 often need both supplemental oxygen and CPAP. In these situations, a split sleep study may be more cost-effective than PM followed by a PSG titration. Most PM devices would miss significant cardiac arrhythmias because typically a heart rate signal derived from the oximeter is recorded rather than ECG. PM is also not indicated in patients in whom other sleep disorders are present that would be better evaluated by PSG (coexistent OSA and parasomnias).

Recommended PM Methodology

The CGPM[26] recommends monitoring at a minimum airflow, respiratory effort, and arterial oxygen saturation (ie, type 3 (III) study) (**Box 8**). The recommended sensors for PM are the same as those recommended for PSG in the AASM scoring manual.[43] PM should be performed under the auspices of an AASM-accredited sleep center. In the recent AASM standards for OCST a greater diversity of monitoring equipment is deemed acceptable (see **Box 8**). Adequately trained personnel should either place the monitoring equipment on the patient or train them on the application of the sensors. The PM data must be viewed in the raw form and, if automated scoring is used, it must be edited for accuracy. For quality assurance, standard operating procedures for the PM process must exist. To verify adequate scoring, inter-rater reliability on scoring of PM studies should be performed on a routine basis and documented. If the PM recording is technically inadequate or if the study results are negative in a patient with a high pretest probability of having OSA, an attended PSG should be performed.

Practical Considerations for PM

In setting up a PM program, there are several technical and economic factors that must be carefully considered for a program to be successful. A system that works in one locale may not work in another. A systematic approach is indicated to avoid a high percentage of technically inadequate PM studies (**Boxes 9** and **10**). The choice of the device and method of device application are major considerations. Devices with more sensors provide more information but are more difficult to apply. Before selecting a PM device, the method of device setup that is planned is an important

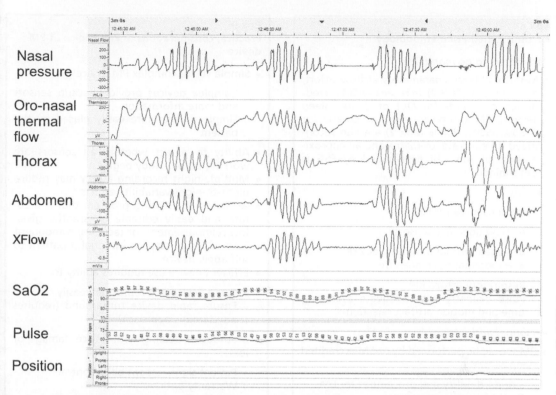

Fig. 4. A 3-minute tracing from a type 3(III) PM device (Embletta) by Embla. The XFlow is a derived signal obtained by taking the derivative of the sum of the thorax and abdominal respiratory inductance plethysmography tracings. Actigraphy was also recorded but is not shown. The illustrated event is a central apnea of the Cheyne-Stokes type.

consideration. The PM device software should provide the ability to review the raw data in detail. Having accurate autoscoring to minimize the amount of event editing that is required is highly desirable given the low reimbursement for the technical component of PM monitoring. If the software is similar to that used for PSG, this may be an advantage to reduce training costs. The durability of the device and cost of expendables (nasal cannula, oximeter probes) should be considered. Devices with a rechargeable battery may help reduce costs because devices using standard batteries typically need a new battery for each patient. The ability of the device to record multiple nights may also be helpful.

PM devices can be placed on the patient in the sleep center or in the home by a technologist (see **Box 10**). However, the application of the PM device by a technologist in private homes is expensive and has safety issues. Therefore, having patients come to a sleep center is recommended if possible. Alternatively, patients can be trained on the PM device and apply the sensors themselves at home. Adequate training is essential and instructional videos or simple instruction sheets can be useful. As noted earlier, one study found more than 3 times

the study failure rate when patients applied PM sensors at home by themselves.[41] One option is to have the patient come to the sleep center for education on device placement and practice sensor application. If patients are unable to successfully attach the sensors, or prefer not to do so, they can simply wear the attached PM device home. PM devices can be returned by the patient to the sleep center or mailed if the commuting distance is long. A rapid turnaround reduces the number of PM devices that need to be purchased. If the PM device is simple, mailing the device to the patient's home with instructions and having them apply the device can work in some patient populations. Device loss can be a major expense. Many sleep centers have patients sign a financial responsibility form stating that they will be charged for lost devices.

There are several common sensor application problems that need to be addressed. Patients often have difficulty applying some types of oximeter probes as well as chest and abdominal belts. The physician should be aware of the options before purchasing a device. During the study at home, dislodgement of either the nasal cannula or oximeter probe, as well as pulling sensor leads out of the PM

Box 8
Recommended PM methodology

Parameters to be monitored

- Monitor at least 3 parameters: airflow, effort, and oximetry (CGPM). In recent AASM accreditation standards for Out of Center Sleep Testing, PM equipment meeting criteria for 95800, 95801, 95806 (**Box 2**) are also recognized if heart rate, oximetry, and an approximation of the AHI determined by PSG is determined.[28]

Sensors

- Same sensors as for PSG
  - Airflow (ideally 2 sensors)
    - Apnea: oronasal thermal device
    - Hypopnea: nasal pressure
  - Respiratory effort: RIP
  - Pulse oximetry with adequate averaging time and motion artifact rejection

Personnel and setting

- PM should be performed by AASM-accredited sleep center
  - Standard policy and procedures for PM
  - Quality assurance program
  - Interscorer reliability program
- Experienced sleep technician/technologist either places sensors or directly educates the patient on sensor application
- Review of raw data and interpretation by BC/BE sleep physician

Device/scoring

- Display of raw data is available for manual scoring and editing
- Scoring criteria according to AASM scoring manual

Follow-up

- If PM study is technically inadequate or fails to establish a diagnosis of OSA in a patient with a high pretest probability, a diagnostic PSG should be performed
- Follow-up visit with MD or trained health care provider following PM testing to discuss results of test with the patient and plan treatment

Abbreviation: BC/BE, board-certified or board-eligible sleep physician.
From Collop NA, Anderson WM, Boehlecke B, et al. Clinical guidelines for the use of unattended portable monitors in the diagnosis of obstructive sleep apnea in adult patients. Portable Monitoring Task Force of the American Academy of Sleep Medicine. J Clin Sleep Med 2007;3:737–47; with permission.

Box 9
Practical considerations in PM: choice of PM device

- Simple versus complex PM device
  - Complex devices provide backup sensors and more information
  - Simple device more easily placed by the patient
- Ability to detect whether all sensors are working before study begins
- Multiple-night recording ability may reduce night-to-night variability effects
- An automatic scoring program that is accurate and easily editable is essential given low reimbursement for technical component
- Ease of device setup is essential if patient to self apply device
- Efficient device use requires ability to:
  - Clean device and reprogram easily
  - Ensure rapid device turnaround (requires a systematic approach)
- Methods of dealing with device damage or loss
  - Patient signs responsibility contract
  - Warranty options
- Software similar to PSG device: less training needed to score studies
- Battery: rechargeable; if not, usually a new battery needed for each study to ensure success
- Body position sensor: helpful with postural OSA

device during body movement, are typical causes of technically inadequate studies. Patients can be trained to apply tape at strategic points to reduce these events. Many devices have the ability to inform the patient and technologist that sensors are working and the device is recording data. For example, some devices use flashing lights or an audible tone to communicate sensor function (or dysfunction). Others provide information the morning after monitoring on the adequacy of data collection, which allows the patient to record another night of data if necessary before returning the device.

It is also useful to have patients complete a brief sleep diary to record their estimate of how long they slept and whether the night of sleep was typical. An occasional patient sleeps poorly with the device attached. If minimal sleep is recorded, a false-negative study is likely. Devices that can record more than 1 night provide another monitoring night opportunity and may also reduce the influence of night-to-night variability.

Box 10
Method of device setup and return

A. *Sleep center setup*

- Advantages

  o Controlled environment
  o Technologist can place device on patient or train patient
  o Patients receive instruction then practice PM setup
  o Patient can wear device home if necessary
  o Individual or group setup

    ▪ Individual PM setup (privacy)
    ▪ Group or class setup (cost savings in personnel time)

- Disadvantages

  o Travel cost for patients (2 round trips unless device mailed back)

B. *In-home setup (technologist travels to home and attaches PM)*

- Advantages

  o Lower % technically inadequate studies (compared with application of sensors and device by patient)

- Disadvantage

  o Travel costs
  o Technologist safety issues

C. *Mail device to patient (return by mail or patient)*

- Requires simple device
- Higher percentage of failed studies

Specific types of PM devices

There are numerous devices available for PM monitoring (**Fig. 5**). This article is not an endorsement of any one device but provides an overview of a few of the more commonly used devices. The CGPM recommend use of the same sensors as for PSG, which mandates the use of both an oronasal thermal device and nasal pressure to monitor airflow and RIP bands to detect respiratory effort. As noted earlier, devices having more sensors provide more information but are more difficult for patients to place. It is always a trade-off between information and complexity of sensor application. Most PM devices monitor airflow using a nasal cannula with monitoring of nasal pressure (with or without a square root transformation). A snoring signal is usually derived from nasal pressure, or a separate snore sensor can be used. Some PM devices can simultaneously record oronasal thermal flow along with nasal pressure. Respiratory effort is typically detected with 1 or more piezoelectric or RIP bands. Some PM devices use reusable effort bands, whereas others have an option of disposable band material. Cleaning of devices between patients is an important consideration as well as the cost of expendables. Sao_2 and pulse rate are typically determined by pulse oximetry. Several oximeter probe options are available including clip or adhesive wrap probes (either reusable or disposable). The reusable adhesive wrap approach is cheaper but more difficult for the patient to apply. Many PM devices also have the capability of recording body position and movement (actigraphy). Actigraphy is used by some devices to exclude portions of the tracing from analysis when there is considerable patient movement.

The Stardust II (Philips Respironics, Murrysville, PA, USA) uses a nasal pressure flow sensor, a piezoelectric effort belt, oximetry, and a body position sensor (see **Fig. 5**). The device is easy for patients to apply. The same company also produces the PDX which has the capability to record more channels of sensor data. A typical setup includes oronasal thermal flow, nasal pressure, thorax and abdominal RIP belts, oximetry, and a body position sensor (see **Fig. 1**). The device can record more than 1 night of data and has the ability to inform the patient of the quality of the previous night's recording.

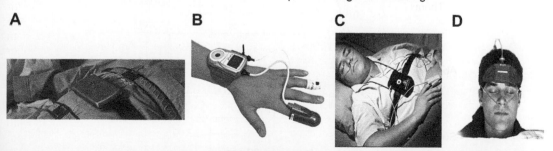

A   **B**   **C**   **D**

Fig. 5. PM devices (*A*) (Embletta, Embla), (*B*) WatchPAT 200 (Itamar), (*C*) Stardust II (Philips Respironics), (*D*) ARES (Watermark Inc.). (Part [A] *courtesy of* Embla, Inc; with permission. Part [B] *courtesy of* Itamar Medical, Inc, Caesarea, Israel; with permission. Part [C] *courtesy of* Phillips Respironics, Murrysville, PA; with permission. Part [D] *courtesy of* Watermark Medical, Inc, Boca Raton, FL; with permission.)

The Embletta® Gold™ (Embla, Denver CO) has many different recording capabilities (see **Fig. 5**). Typically nasal pressure, thorax and abdominal respiratory effort (RIP), oximetry, and body position are recorded. There is the option to record or-onasal thermal flow and differential pressure. The device has built in actigraphy and this assists in eliminating periods of wake from the analysis. A unique option is the ability of the device to derive an estimate of flow from the RIP band signals (**Fig. 4**). Basically, the RIPsum of the thorax and abdominal effort bands is derived (an estimate of tidal volume). Then the time derivative of the RIP-sum is computed and this is an estimate of airflow (Xflow®) which is displayed as a signal. The XFlow signal is useful if the nasal pressure cannula or or-onasal devices are dislodged during the study or not available (**Fig. 6**). The downside of using two RIP belts is that they may be more difficult for the patient to place than a single effort belt used in some other devices. Use of a single belt does provide less information but may be sufficient in some patients.

The Apnea-Risk Evaluation System Unicorder (ARES) (Watermark Medical, Boca Raton, FL) is a unique PM device (see **Fig. 5D**)[30,44] positioned on the head, and does not require additional wires to external devices. The ARES device measures oxygen saturation, pulse rate, airflow, respiratory effort, snoring levels, head movement, and head position from a wireless recorder self-applied with a single strap to the forehead.

Reflectance oximetry is used to obtain the Spo_2 and pulse rate signals. Airflow is obtained via a nasal cannula and a pressure transducer. A calibrated acoustic microphone is used to acquire quantified snoring levels (dB). Accelerometers are used to measure head movement and derive head position. The recorder was designed to be easily affixed by the patient, and provide alerts during the study if poor quality airflow or Spo_2 is detected so the device could be adjusted. The device also has the ability to record EEG from electrodes on the forehead (FP1 and FP2; estimate of sleep) and can record multiple nights of data.

PAT

Unique PM devices are available that detect respiratory events by recording changes in sympathetic tone (rather than airflow) using PAT.[45–50] The devices using this technology (WatchPAT 100,200, Itamar Medial) are worn on the wrist. The devices haves 2 probes: a PAT probe and an oximetry probe worn on separate digits. The PAT signal is a measure of the blood volume in the digit. When sympathetic tone increases, stimulation of α receptors causes vasoconstriction of the blood vessels in the digit, which decreases fingertip volume and the PAT signal. As surges in sympathetic tone follow respiratory event termination, the combination of a decrease in PAT signal, a decrease in Spo_2 followed by an increase, and an increase in heart rate allow determination of respiratory events (**Fig. 7**).

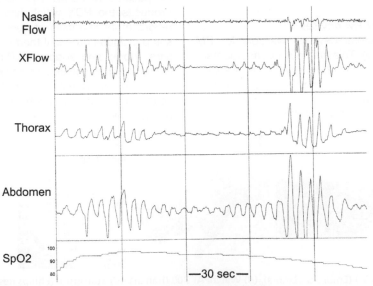

Fig. 6. In this tracing from an Embletta, the nasal flow channel is inadequate (likely nasal cannula dislodged or occluded) but the derived XFlow (time derivative of sum of the thorax and abdomen RIP bands signals) provides a reasonable estimate of flow and can be used to score respiratory events.

Nonrespiratory arousals would not reduce the Spo2. The device has built-in actigraphy and novel algorithms designed for patients with sleep apnea to help with estimation of sleep.[48] Recently, the combination of actigraphy and the PAT signal has been used to determine estimates of wake, light and deep non-REM (NREM) sleep, and REM sleep because the sympathetic tone characteristics of these sleep stages differ.[49] An optional combined body position and snore sensor can be placed on the sternum. The PAT devices have been well validated by studies comparing the results with PSG. The results include an AHI and RDI based on estimated TST. The device is one of the easier PM devices to apply. The device cannot be used in patients on α-blockers (eg, terazosin) and with patients in atrial fibrillation. Another downside is that the PAT probes are expensive. The NCD for HST[12] recognizes 3 channels of monitoring including PAT, oximetry, and actigraphy as a valid PM method. However, PAT studies are not reimbursed in all locales. PAT devices are not within the recommended CGPM device guidelines but are acceptable by new AASM standards for OCST provided a reasonable estimate of the AHI (RDI) can be determined. The raw data are available for viewing and editing. However, the algorithm for identification of respiratory events is proprietary and editing of events is problematic. A reviewer can assess the technical adequacy of recorded data.

Type 4 (IV) Devices

This article focuses on type 3 (III) devices but type IV devices including oximetry are useful in some situations. The devices can be used to identify patients at high risk for having OSA (ie, before other definitive testing). CMS defines type IV devices as those measuring at least 3 channels of data, one of which is airflow. The CGPM did not recommend type IV PM devices. However, type IV devices may meet criteria for the 95801 procedure code, and if so are acceptable in the AASM OCST standards. An example of a popular single-channel monitor is the ApneaLink (ResMed, Poway, CA, USA). This device can be used in the single-channel mode (nasal pressure and derived snoring) or in the dual-sensor mode with oximetry.[51,52] Several outcome studies[36,37] used oximetry to select a high-probability group of patients OSA. Simpler devices require less expertise in application and may be easier for patient application at home.

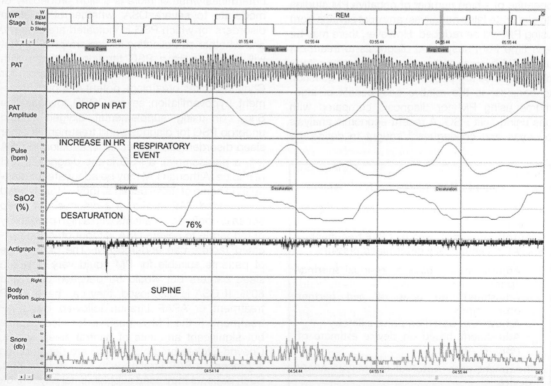

Fig. 7. PAT detection of a respiratory event. The PAT signal decreases (increased sympathetic tone) associated with an increase then decrease in pulse and an arterial oxygen desaturation.

Integration of PM Monitoring into an Overall Patient Care Algorithm

Diagnosis of OSA using PM is only the first part of the process if the study is positive. It is expected, in populations with a high probability of OSA, that a high percentage of PM tests will be positive. If PAP is chosen for treatment, there are several alternative pathways to proceed (**Box 11**). The standard approach would be to perform a PSG PAP titration and subsequent PAP treatment. Patients could also use an Auto-PAP device at home (typically for 3 or more nights), and information obtained could be used to select a pressure for chronic CPAP treatment (autotitration, using 90 or 95th percentile pressure).[37–39,53] A third possible approach is starting CPAP at a pressure derived using prediction equations, with subsequent adjustment based on oximetry, symptoms, or machine estimates of the residual AHI.[53–55] A fourth approach is simply to treat patients with an Auto-CPAP (auto-adjusting PAP device [APAP]). This eliminates the need for PSG or auto-CPAP titration) and reduces the time from diagnosis to treatment.

Issues of cost and reimbursement vary between settings (VA Health Care System versus private sector). If a large number of PM studies are technically inadequate or if PSG must be performed because of a high number of negative PM studies (to eliminate false negatives) any cost savings from using PM will be reduced. However, there may be less time from suspected diagnosis to treatment using PM clinical pathways. If a high percentage of PM studies are positive, a reasonable question to consider is the relative cost-benefit of algorithms using PM for diagnosis compared with one using split PSG. A recent economic analysis by Ayas and colleagues[56] sought to define the pretest probability of OSA needed for PM studies to be cost-effective. Compared with use of diagnostic PSG (followed by PSG titration), the probability was 0.47 and, compared with split studies, the pretest probability was 0.68. This study illustrates that PM offers less economic advantages when split studies are frequently performed.

In the private sector, autotitration studies are not reimbursed. If a patient was simply started on APAP treatment, a PAP titration would not be necessary in many cases. However, the cost of an APAP device exceeds that for CPAP, whereas DME companies receive the same reimbursement from insurance providers for both types of devices. These facts currently limit the use of alternatives to PSG titration. Thus, most patients diagnosed with OSA by PM in the private sector currently need a PSG titration However, if the cost differential between APAP and CPAP units for DME providers continues to decrease, the option of APAP treatment will be more financially viable. It is also possible that insurance providers may someday be willing to provide additional reimbursement for APAP devices rather than pay for a PSG titration.

Overall Approach to Using PSG and PM

An overall approach to using a combination of PSG and PM is presented in **Fig. 8**. A clinical evaluation determines whether there is a high probability of moderate to severe OSA, whether other sleep disorders for which PSG is indicated are present, and whether complicating issues are present that will likely require a PSG titration. Patients with moderate to severe CHF (a risk factor for Cheyne-Stokes breathing), potent narcotics treatment, hypoventilation, severe COPD, low baseline SaO_2, or using supplemental oxygen should undergo PSG for diagnosis and treatment. If other sleep disorders are suspected in addition to OSA (eg, a parasomnia), a PSG is the diagnostic test of choice. Although PM may be adequate for diagnosis in some of these patients, they will likely need an attended PAP titration if a diagnosis of sleep apnea is confirmed. Patients with a high probability of moderate to severe OSA without other complicated factors can undergo PM. The percentage of patients suitable for PM could vary between sleep centers but would be between 50% and 80%. If OSA is diagnosed, they can have APAP treatment or APAP titration followed by CPAP treatment. If the PM is positive for sleep apnea but significant amounts of central sleep apnea, Cheyne-Stokes breathing, or severe desaturation is present, a PAP titration with PSG is indicated. Such patients may need supplemental oxygen, bilevel PAP, or PAP mode with a backup rate. If the

---

Box 11
PAP treatment after PM diagnosis of OSA

- PSG PAP titration followed by CPAP treatment
- Autotitration followed by CPAP treatment
- CPAP on empirically determined pressure

  o Adjustment on basis of residual snoring/apnea

  o Adjustment on basis of bed partner observations

  o Adjustment based on pulse oximetry

  o Adjustment based on device estimate of residual AHI

- Treatment with AutoPAP (autoCPAP, APAP) device

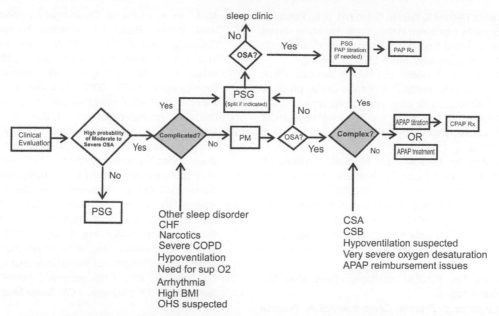

Fig. 8. Possible algorithm for use of PM. Patients with high probability of moderate to severe OSA and no complicating factors undergo a PM. If OSA is diagnosed, the PM findings are used to triage the patient to PSG titration or alternative pathways using autotitrating PAP. Patients with central apnea or severe oxygen desaturation would undergo PSG titration. APAP, auto positive airway pressure; COPD, chronic obstructive pulmonary disease; CSA, central sleep apnea; CSB, Cheyne-Stokes Breathing; OHS, obesity hypoventilation syndrome, Rx, treatment.

PM is negative, a PSG can be performed. The initial clinical evaluation is used to triage patients to PM or PSG and the results of the PM study are used to triage patients to PSG, PSG PAP titration, APAP titration, or APAP treatment.

SUMMARY

Portable sleep monitoring will likely play an increasingly important role in sleep medicine. Like all diagnostic tools, PM requires expertise in selecting patients to be studied, proper interpretation of results, and decision making concerning the need for treatment or other diagnostic studies. Technology is expected to improve so that portable monitors are easier to place and are less cumbersome and more reliable. Although some have viewed PM as a threat to traditional PSG, PM has many limitations. Many patients with OSA and comorbidities will continue to benefit from PSG for diagnosis and PAP titration. However, PM may help identify many patients with OSA who would otherwise have gone undiagnosed and untreated.

REFERENCES

1. Indications for Polysomnography Task Force ASDA. Practice parameters for the indications for polysomnography and related procedures. Sleep 1997;20:406–22.
2. Chesson AL Jr, Ferber RA, Fry JM, et al. The indications for polysomnography and related procedures. A Standard of Practice Review. Sleep 1997;20:423–87.
3. Kushida CA, Littner MR, Morgenthaler T, et al. Practice parameters for the indications for polysomnography and related procedures: an update for 2005. Sleep 2005;28:499–521.
4. Littner MR. Portable monitoring in the diagnosis of the obstructive sleep apnea syndrome. Semin Respir Crit Care Med 2005;26:56–67.
5. Gay PC, Selecky PA. Are sleep studies appropriately done in the home? Respir Care 2010;55:66–75.
6. Flemons WW, Douglas NJ, Kuna ST, et al. Access to diagnosis and treatment of patients with suspected sleep apnea. Am J Respir Crit Care Med 2004; 169:668–72.
7. Ferber R, Millman R, Coppola M, et al. Portable recording in the assessment of obstructive sleep apnea. ASDA Standards of Practice. Sleep 1994;17:378–92.
8. Flemons WW, Littner MR, Rowley JA, et al. Home diagnosis of sleep apnea: a systematic review of the literature. An evidence review cosponsored by the American Academy of Sleep Medicine, the American College of Chest Physicians, and the American Thoracic Society. Chest 2003;124:1543–79.
9. Quan SF, Howard BV, Iber C, et al. The Sleep Heart Health Study: design, rationale, and methods. Sleep 1997;20:1077–85.

10. Iber C, Redline S, Kaplan Gilpin AM, et al. Polysomnography performed in the unattended home versus the attended laboratory setting–Sleep Heart Health Study methodology. Sleep 2004;27:536–40.

11. Department of Health and Human Services. Decision memo for continuous positive airway pressure (CPAP) therapy for obstructive sleep apnea (OSA). CAG#0093R. Available at: http://wwwcmshhsgov/mcd/viewdecisionmemoasp?id=204. Accessed November 1, 2010.

12. Centers for Medicare and Medicaid Services M, 2009. Decision memo for sleep testing for obstructive sleep apnea (CAG-00405N). Available at: http://wwwcmshhsgov/mcd/viewdecisionmemoasp?id_227. Accessed November 1, 2010.

13. Collop NA. Portable monitoring for the diagnosis of obstructive sleep apnea. Curr Opin Pulm Med 2008;14:525–9.

14. Collop NA. Portable monitoring. Sleep Med Clin 2009;4:435–42.

15. Standards of Practice Committee ASDA. Practice parameters for the use of portable recording in the assessment of obstructive sleep apnea. Sleep 1994;17:372–7.

16. Ross SD, Sheinhait IA, Harrison KJ, et al. Systematic review and meta-analysis of the literature regarding the diagnosis of sleep apnea. Sleep 2000;23:519–32.

17. Chesson AL Jr, Berry RB, Pack A. Practice parameters for the use of portable monitoring devices in the investigation of suspected obstructive sleep apnea in adults. Sleep 2003;26:907–13.

18. ATS/ACCP/AASM Portable Monitoring Taskforce Steering Committee. Executive summary on the systematic review and practice parameters for portable monitoring in the investigation of suspected sleep apnea in adults. Am J Respir Crit Care Med 2004;169:1160–3.

19. Davidson T. A request to reassess the national coverage determination for diagnosis and treatment of obstructive sleep apnea (OSA) to include multichannel home sleep testing as an alternative to polysomnography (PSG). 2004. Available at: http://wwwcmsgov/DeterminationProcess/downloads/id110pdf. Accessed November 1, 2010.

20. Agency for Healthcare Research and Quality (submitted by RTI). Effectiveness of portable monitoring devices for diagnosing obstructive sleep apnea: update of a systematic review. 2004. Available at: http://wwwcmsgov/determinationprocess/downloads/id24TApdf. Accessed November 1, 2010.

21. Centers for Medicare and Medicaid Services. Decision memo for continuous positive airway pressure (CPAP) therapy for obstructive sleep apnea (OSA) (CAG-00093R). 2005. Available at: http://wwwcmsgov/mcd/viewdecisionmemoasp?id=110. Accessed November 1, 2010.

22. American Academy of Otolaryngology-Head and Neck Surgery. Request to reassess the National Coverage Determination (NCD) for diagnosis and treatment of obstructive sleep apnea (OSA) to include home sleep testing as an alternative to polysomnography (PSG). 2007. Available at: http://wwwcmsgov/determinationprocess/downloads/id204pdf. Accessed November 1, 2010.

23. Agency for Healthcare Research and Quality. Technology assessment: home diagnosis of obstructive sleep apnea-hypopnea syndrome. 2007. Available at: http://wwwcmshhsgov/determinationprocess/downloads/id48TApdf. Accessed November 1, 2010.

24. Agency for Healthcare Research and Quality. Obstructive sleep apnea-hypopnea syndrome: modeling different diagnostic strategies. 2007. Available at: http://wwwcmshhsgov/determinationprocess/downloads/id50TApdf. Accessed November 1, 2010.

25. Chediak AD. Why CMS approved home sleep testing for CPAP coverage. J Clin Sleep Med 2008;4:16–8.

26. Collop NA, Anderson WM, Boehlecke B, et al. Clinical guidelines for the use of unattended portable monitors in the diagnosis of obstructive sleep apnea in adult patients. Portable Monitoring Task Force of the American Academy of Sleep Medicine. J Clin Sleep Med 2007;3:737–47.

27. Centers for Medicare and Medicaid Services M, 2009. Proposed decision memo for continuous positive airway pressure (CPAP) therapy for obstructive sleep apnea (OSA). CAG#0093R2. Available at: https://wwwcmsgov/scripts/ctredirectordll/pdf?@_CPR0a0a043a07d1KA_Whnn_4XYw. Accessed November 1, 2010.

28. Available at: http://www.aasmnet.org/resources/pdf/OCSTstandards.pdf. Assessed June 16, 2011.

29. Dingli K, Coleman EL, Vennelle M, et al. Evaluation of a portable device for diagnosing the sleep apnoea/hypopnoea syndrome. Eur Respir J 2003;21:253–9.

30. Levendowski D, Steward D, Woodson BT, et al. The impact of obstructive sleep apnea variability measured in-lab versus in-home on sample size calculations. Int Arch Med 2009;2:2.

31. Smith LA, Chong DW, Vennelle M, et al. Diagnosis of sleep-disordered breathing in patients with chronic heart failure: evaluation of a portable limited sleep study system. J Sleep Res 2007;16:428–35.

32. Flemons WW, Littner MR. Measuring agreement between diagnostic devices. Chest 2003;124:1535–42.

33. Santos-Silva R, Sartori DE, Truksinas V, et al. Validation of a portable monitoring system for the diagnosis of obstructive sleep apnea syndrome. Sleep 2009;32:629–36.

34. Calleja JM, Esnaola S, Rubio R, et al. Comparison of a cardiorespiratory device versus polysomnography for diagnosis of sleep apnoea. Eur Respir J 2002;20:1505–10.

35. Bland JM, Altman DG. Measuring agreement in method comparison studies. Stat Methods Med Res 1999;8:135–60.

36. Whitelaw WA, Brant RF, Flemons WW. Clinical usefulness of home oximetry compared with polysomnography for assessment of sleep apnea. Am J Respir Crit Care Med 2005;171:188–93.

37. Mulgrew AT, Fox N, Ayas NT, et al. Diagnosis and initial management of obstructive sleep apnea without polysomnography: a randomized validation study. Ann Intern Med 2007;146:157–66.

38. Berry RB, Hill G, Thompson L, et al. Portable monitoring and autotitration versus polysomnography for the diagnosis and treatment of sleep apnea. Sleep 2008;31:1423–31.

39. Antic NA, Buchan C, Esterman A, et al. A randomized controlled trial of nurse-led care for symptomatic moderate-severe obstructive sleep apnea. Am J Respir Crit Care Med 2009;179:501–8.

40. Skomro RP, Gjevre J, Reid J, et al. Outcomes of home-based diagnosis and treatment of obstructive sleep apnea. Chest 2010;138:257–63.

41. Golpe R, Jimenez A, Carpizo R. Home sleep studies in the assessment of sleep apnea/hypopnea syndrome. Chest 2002;122:1156–61.

42. Kushida CA, Morgenthaler TI, Littner MR, et al. Practice parameters for the treatment of snoring and obstructive sleep apnea with oral appliances: an update for 2005. Sleep 2006;29:240–3.

43. Iber C, Ancoli-Israel S, Chesson AS, et al. The AASM manual for the scoring of sleep and associated events: rules, terminology and technical specification. Westchester (IL): American Academy of Sleep Medicine; 2007.

44. Ayappa I, Norman RG, Seelall V, et al. Validation of a self-applied unattended monitor for sleep disordered breathing. J Clin Sleep Med 2008;4:26–37.

45. Bar A, Pillar G, Dvir I, et al. Evaluation of a portable device based on peripheral arterial tone for unattended home sleep studies. Chest 2003;123:695–703.

46. Pillar G, Bar A, Betito M, et al. An automatic ambulatory device for detection of AASM defined arousals from sleep: the WP100. Sleep Med 2003; 4:207–12.

47. Ayas NT, Pittman S, MacDonald M, et al. Assessment of a wrist-worn device in the detection of obstructive sleep apnea. Sleep Med 2003;4:435–42.

48. Hedner J, Pillar G, Pittman SD, et al. A novel adaptive wrist actigraphy algorithm for sleep-wake assessment in sleep apnea patients. Sleep 2004; 27:1560–6.

49. Herscovici S, Pe'er A, Papyan S, et al. Detecting REM sleep from the finger: an automatic REM sleep algorithm based on peripheral arterial tone (PAT) and actigraphy. Physiol Meas 2007;28:129–40.

50. Choi JH, Kim EJ, Kim YS, et al. Validation study of portable device for the diagnosis of obstructive sleep apnea according to the new AASM scoring criteria: Watch-PAT 100. Acta Otolaryngol 2010; 130:838–43.

51. Erman MK, Stewart D, Einhorn D, et al. Validation of the ApneaLink for the screening of sleep apnea: a novel and simple single-channel recording device. J Clin Sleep Med 2007;3:387–92.

52. Rice TB, Dunn RE, Lincoln AE, et al. Sleep-disordered breathing in the National Football League. Sleep 2010;33:819–24.

53. Masa JF, Jimenez A, Duran J, et al. Alternative methods of titrating continuous positive airway pressure: a large multicenter study. Am J Respir Crit Care Med 2004;170:1218–24.

54. Fitzpatrick MF, Alloway CE, Wakeford TM, et al. Can patients with obstructive sleep apnea titrate their own continuous positive airway pressure? Am J Respir Crit Care Med 2003;167:716–22.

55. Desai H, Patel A, Patel P, et al. Accuracy of auto-titrating CPAP to estimate the residual apnea-hypopnea index in patients with obstructive sleep apnea on treatment with auto-titrating CPAP. Sleep Breath 2009;13:383–90.

56. Ayas NT, Fox J, Epstein L, et al. Initial use of portable monitoring versus polysomnography to confirm obstructive sleep apnea in symptomatic patients: an economic decision model. Sleep Med 2010;11:320–4.

Use of Portable Monitoring for Sleep-Disordered Breathing Treated with an Oral Appliance

Dennis R. Bailey, DDS[a,b,*]

KEYWORDS

- Oral appliances • Portable monitoring • Home sleep study
- Screening • Titration

The potential use of a portable monitor to assess the outcome of treatment with an oral appliance would ideally be performed by the dentist who is managing the patient's sleep-disordered breathing. A sleep medicine physician or sleep center may also perform such a study. The dentist may be using portable monitoring as a means of assessing the response to the oral appliance after an initial titration period along with assessment of the patient's symptom resolution before referral back to the patient's physician, sleep medicine specialist, or for a follow-up polysomnogram. Portable monitoring may be one of the most cost-effective ways for the treating dentist to assess the outcome or effect of the oral appliance, to determine if further adjustment/modification to the appliance is needed, and to retest to determine the current status following any adjustment or modification.

This article emphasizes the use of portable monitors primarily for follow-up care and assessment as opposed to diagnosis or, as it is sometimes referred to, screening. Many have advocated the use of portable monitor type devices as a means by which the dentist can screen patients who might be at risk for sleep apnea.[1,2] This is clearly a diagnostic procedure for a potential medical condition that is not within the scope of dental practice at

this time. Portable monitors, specifically level 3 devices, have limited use as an alternative to the overnight polysomnogram (level 1) as an effective instrument for the diagnosis of sleep apnea.[3]

HISTORY AND CURRENT STATUS: A CASE REPORT

A 54-year old man presents to a dentist who has advanced training and is competent in dental sleep medicine and the use of oral appliances for managing sleep-disordered breathing. He was referred to the dentist by the sleep center where the polysomnogram was done and his primary care physician, mainly because he was unable to tolerate continuous positive airway pressure (CPAP) despite trying numerous masks. He had a consultation with an otolaryngologist about possible surgery and was also informed that an oral appliance would be more appropriate at this time. His Epworth Sleepiness Scale score was 13 (the normal value is >10) and the apnea/hypopnea index (AHI) was 21 per hour of sleep. His body mass index is 28 kg/m^2 and his neck size is 40 cm. He has been diagnosed with hypertension, which is controlled with Lisinopril and hydrochlorothiazide. With medication, his blood pressure is 121/82. He denies having any other health-related

[a] Orofacial Pain and Dental Sleep Medicine Department, UCLA School of Dentistry, Los Angeles, CA, USA
[b] Dental Sleep Mini-Residency, UCLA School of Dentistry, Los Angeles, CA, USA
* 8400 East Prentice Avenue, Suite 804, Greenwood Village, CO 80111.
E-mail address: RMC4E@aol.com

Sleep Med Clin 6 (2011) 335–340
doi:10.1016/j.jsmc.2011.05.012
1556-407X/11/$ – see front matter © 2011 Elsevier Inc. All rights reserved.

issues, specifically cardiovascular disease or diabetes. He reports that his sleep onset is within 15 minutes but his sleep is restless with multiple awakenings (2–3 per night) and he gets 6 hours of sleep a night on average. He reports that he has snored for more than 20 years; and in the last 5 years the snoring has become more problematic and observed apnea has occurred.

A formal orofacial and airway evaluation was performed as has been described and recommended for the dentist who performs this type of service.[4] This also included an evaluation of the nasal airway. During the evaluation, he denied being a mouth breather at night and has no difficulty breathing through the nose. However, nasal dilation (commonly known as the Cottle test) improved the patient's ability to nose breath. He did report trying nasal strips for nasal dilation but they were not effective for the snoring and did not seem to affect his sleep.

By virtue of testing, it was determined that with the mandible repositioned, which included opening the vertical approximately 5 mm and advancing the mandible 2–3 mm, he believed his airway was improved and he would not snore. At this point, an oral appliance was determined to be an appropriate treatment and the necessary records were obtained for the fabrication of the oral appliance.

At the first follow-up 2 weeks after receiving the oral appliance, he reports that the snoring is significantly improved, he feels his sleep and feeling of being tired and sleepy during the day are improved. He also feels he is more productive at work and not as tired at the end of the day. Some adjustment to the oral appliance is done mainly for comfort and he is reappointed in a month. He has had the oral appliance for 6 weeks and reports that his symptoms continue to improve and his snoring is present but much improved. Because of the snoring, his mandible is advanced approximately 2 mm and with this change he feels his breathing is also improved. He is reappointed for a follow-up visit in another month.

At the third follow-up visit he reports that the snoring is no longer present according to his wife and he continues to believe that he has improved energy levels and is sleeping through the night. He awakens rested and wakes up without an alarm most mornings. By report, his initial complaints and neurocognitive symptoms are improved (**Table 1**). At this point no further adjustment is deemed necessary and he is reappointed for a follow-up visit in 2 months.

He has now had the oral appliance for more than 4 months and is satisfied with the results. At this time a portable monitoring sleep study to assess the effect of the oral appliance and to determine if

Table 1
Case report: symptoms of obstructive sleep apnea before and after use of an oral appliance

Symptom	Before Oral Appliance Use	With Oral Appliance Use
Snoring	Present	Resolved
Epworth Sleepiness Scale score	13	5
Excessive daytime sleepiness	Present	Reduced/ improved
Drowsy driving	Present	Eliminated
Concentration	Difficult	Improved
Energy levels	Low	Improved/ resolved
Observed apnea	Present at times	None
Mood swings/irritable	Present	Resolved
Restless sleep	Present	Resolved
Awakenings each night	2 to 3	None now
Headaches	Occasional (2–3 a week)	None

any further adjustment is needed, is arranged. It is explained that this is not the same type of sleep study that he had initially. This study is not for diagnosis of sleep apnea (this has already been done) but to determine if the appliance is managing the apnea adequately. The appropriate consent forms are completed and he is scheduled to have the study done.

The portable monitoring study is completed after the patient is instructed on the use and application of the equipment. He will do a 1-night study and return the equipment to the office the next day. At that time, the data will be downloaded for review. The results of the portable monitoring study reveal that the AHI is now 7 and his blood oxygen levels are in the 90% or greater range, nearly 100% of the time. His Epworth Sleepiness Scale score is now 5. At this time he seems to be deriving a reasonable outcome with the oral appliance. A report is generated and will be sent to the referring physician, to the sleep center where the initial sleep study was performed, and to any other physicians who are directly involved with the patient's care. A decision will be made regarding the need for an attended level 1 sleep study to further substantiate the effect of the oral appliance and his current level of apnea.

Portable Monitoring for Diagnosis Before Oral Appliance Therapy

The dental sleep medicine practitioner is the one who will most likely be providing an oral appliance. However, the use of portable monitoring to screen for sleep-disordered breathing in those patients who may be at risk for sleep apnea is not within the scope of practice by the dentist. Despite the advanced training the dentist may have in sleep medicine, they, like most primary care physicians, are not well-versed in the recognition of coexisting sleep disorders that may present as the same type of symptoms as sleep-disordered breathing.[5] Even with advanced training, the level 3 portable monitor will not provide adequate information to allow for the diagnosis of comorbid sleep disorders such as central sleep apnea, periodic limb movements (PLMs), parasomnias, various circadian rhythm sleep disorders, or narcolepsy. In addition, the portable monitor is not indicated for use as a general screening device in an asymptomatic population. The more appropriate action is to identify those patients who are at risk for sleep-disordered breathing. Once it is established that the patient is at risk, the patient should be referred to their primary care physician or to a sleep center for a polysomnogram.

In general, the use of the level 3 portable monitor is not accepted as the optimal method for diagnosing sleep-disordered breathing at the present time. The gold standard continues to be the overnight polysomnogram.[3] However, there are numerous articles that support the use of these portable monitors for patients with high pretest probability of being at risk for sleep-disordered breathing.[6,7]

The main issue is that the sensitivity and specificity of these devices at an AHI less than 15 is not as good compared with an AHI greater than 15. One study did find that portable monitoring was most reliable at an AHI of 10 or more.[8] In addition, portable monitors may actually underestimate the severity of sleep apnea. This is related to the computation of the AHI and more specifically, the respiratory disturbance index (RDI) per hour of recording time because of the difference in total sleep time versus total recording time.[9]

Another issue related to diagnosis using a portable monitor, even if it is being used to assess just snoring, is if the outcome is negative (RDI >5), then the patient may not seek or obtain treatment. Who then assumes the liability for the medical consequences of the sleep apnea? Given that the portable monitor may underestimate the degree of sleep apnea, this is of particular concern in patients who are asymptomatic and may only perceive the issue as snoring, not sleep apnea.

The role of the dentist, regardless of the level of training, is to perform risk assessment for a sleep-disordered breathing condition. Risk assessment is initially done by having an awareness of the following[4]:

1. Assessment of findings through questions in the health history (screening)
2. Assessment of the most common symptoms of sleep-disordered breathing
3. Awareness of existing medical conditions that indicate the possible risk for sleep-disordered breathing
4. Use of standard questionnaires such as the Epworth Sleepiness Scale or the Berlin questionnaire
5. Findings from the head/oral/airway clinical evaluation.

Based on the assessment of risk and comorbid conditions, the patient is referred to a sleep medicine specialist or for a sleep study. That study would most likely be a polysomnogram.

Portable Monitoring for Progressive/Follow-Up Testing with Oral Appliance Therapy

The use of level 3 portable monitoring based on published clinical guidelines has been recommended (consensus) for the purpose of determining the effectiveness of oral appliance therapy for sleep-disordered breathing.[3] This is stated as follows:

Sect 1.4 PM: "Portable Monitoring (PM) may be indicted to monitor the response to non-CPAP treatments for obstructive sleep apnea, including oral appliances, upper airway surgery, and weight loss."

Furthermore, the use of level 3 portable monitors for assessment of the effectiveness of an oral appliance after the final adjustment is a practice parameter guideline.[10] A more practical point of view would potentially use the portable monitor at various points in the titration process of the treatment to determine if added adjustment or modification is needed before a more definitive sleep study. Assuming that the level 3 portable monitor is reliable, its use would contribute to improvement in consistent and successful use of the oral appliance for the management of sleep apnea.[8] In some cases, the level 3 portable monitoring study may actually be satisfactory in determining that the oral appliance is adequately addressing the sleep-disordered breathing. This is a decision that ultimately should be made by the sleep medicine specialist, not the treating dentist.

The American Academy of Dental Sleep Medicine (AADSM) in 2005 also established a position as it relates to the use of portable monitoring.[11] The position that has been taken is that the use of portable monitoring should be restricted to use for titration of the oral appliance (the need for adjustment and modification) for an enhanced effect and to document the effectiveness of the treatment. Furthermore, the use of portable monitors "as a screening tool" designed to identify those patients who may require an overnight polysomnogram is not endorsed at this time. In 2009, the AADSM published a treatment protocol for oral appliances that indicated that portable monitoring was applicable for gathering objective data for the purpose of oral appliance titration.[12]

Based on studies that have looked at the use of level 3 portable monitors compared with polysomnograms for diagnosis, it seems that the portable monitor should provide information to determine that the oral appliance is adequately resolving the sleep-disordered breathing and has also improved the patient's symptoms. Concern for the recognition of other coexisting sleep disorders is not an issue with the use of this technology because these conditions have most likely been recognized (diagnosed) from the original polysomnogram and their management is being considered aside from the use of the oral appliance for the sleep-disordered breathing. Consequently, not all of the parameters of the sleep study are needed to ascertain that the oral appliance is effectively managing the sleep-disordered breathing. The parameters of greatest value in evaluating the effectiveness of the oral appliance are listed in **Table 2**.

Assessment of the AHI based on the use of a thermistor may underestimate the number of hypopneas.[13] Measurement of nasal pressure is more sensitive but may be subject to signal loss. More importantly, mouth breathing will also decrease the effectiveness of this measuring device. The presence of mouth breathing in patients with sleep apnea is a significant issue that is often underevaluated and insufficiently addressed. Before any testing using the portable monitor, an effort should be made to address mouth breathing when using an oral appliance and strategies should be used to improve the nasal airway and nasal breathing while using the appliance. This is best done using nasal rinses, nasal dilation, and in some cases, nasal airway surgery. Myofunctional tongue therapy has also been shown to be helpful with improvement of the tongue posture and by achieving a lip seal, which may improve nasal breathing during sleep.[14] If the patient continues

Table 2
Parameters of value to determine effectiveness of an oral appliance with portable monitoring

Parameter Being Tested	Significance
AHI	Needs to be less than 10 and ideally less than 5 (not always possible due to sensitivity and specificity for ≤ 10 or ≤ 15) based on the device
Snoring	Need to evaluate presence or resolution If present, for what period of time
Oxygen saturation	Ideally needs to be in the 90% range nearly 100% of the time Need to distinguish parameter of desaturation (3% vs 4%)
Sleep position	Not always available on all devices
Sleep bruxism (optional)	Ideal from the standpoint of the dentist and as a coexisting condition Not available on portable monitors; can be adapted on selected devices

to be predominately a mouth breather, this needs to be considered when the level 3 portable monitor is being used for titration. In this type of situation, the oral appliance should be titrated to an optimum outcome and the patient should have an overnight polysomnogram to better ascertain the effectiveness of the oral appliance.

A poster presentation at the AADSM annual meeting in June 2010 addressed the use of portable monitoring (home sleep monitoring) for the purpose of guiding the titration of the oral appliance. The study looked at 32 subjects who had been diagnosed with moderate to severe sleep apnea. The testing device reported the AHI, the amount of time that the oxygen saturation was less than 90% and the O_2 nadir.[15] By using such a system it was determined that the oral appliance was effective in 71% of the patients. It was also found that the O_2 nadir increased by 4.5% and the percent of time the oxygen saturation was less than 90% improved by 64%. This was also correlated to the patient's symptoms; there was a significant improvement in quality of life and daytime sleepiness was improved in 90% of the patients in the study. The conclusion here is that once the patient has experienced a subjective improvement in the initial symptoms, the portable monitor can be used to determine if there is also improvement objectively.

When the results of the portable monitoring testing are found to be satisfactory, there should also be adequate resolution of the symptoms that were present before the use of the oral appliance. When symptoms continue to be present, it may be due to other coexisting sleep disorders and not due to the sleep-disordered breathing. This is possibly the case with conditions such as sleep bruxism, insomnia, and PLM disorder. In these cases, the portable monitoring data may indicate improvement of the sleep apnea, which requires the investigation of other coexisting sleep disorders, often requiring a referral to the sleep medicine specialist.

The use of the portable monitor offers advantages that allow for ongoing assessment of the impact of the oral appliance that cannot be assessed through simple questioning of the patient. By testing at various intervals in the treatment/titration process, the oral appliance can be adjusted and modified based on both subjective as well as objective data. In addition, the issue of improving the nasal airway during sleep can be ongoing in an effort to minimize or eliminate any mouth breathing, and as that therapy progresses the portable monitor will be able to assess the impact on the sleep apnea and how well the oral appliance is performing.

Advantages to use of the level 3 portable monitor include:

1. Ease of use by both the patient and the doctor
2. Cost-effective for determination of the need for oral appliance adjustment and modification (titration)
3. Testing can be done on multiple occasions to allow for ongoing titration of the oral appliance before a more detailed sleep study
4. Results of the study are quickly available.

Disadvantages to use of the level 3 portable monitor include:

1. A lead may come loose and data are lost or not recorded
2. Device may simply not record properly
3. Device may be turned off or be taken off during sleep and thus there are no data recorded
4. Cost of disposables may be a factor in the per test cost
5. Patient may have difficulty hooking up the portable monitor.

The assessment of the successful effect of the oral appliance using portable monitoring may not be totally accurate based on the limitations of these devices as well as the specific limitations of the patient and of coexisting sleep disorders. For these reasons, the outcome of the level 3 portable monitoring study should be shared with the sleep medicine specialist and the patient's primary care physician. The clinical guidelines indicate that when level 3 portable monitors are being used for diagnosis, the results need to be interpreted by a sleep medicine specialist. However, when these same devices are being used for titration, the need for interpreting the results is not defined. At this point, the resolution of the validity of this would best be achieved by a clinical study where an oral appliance is being used that compares the simultaneous use of the level 3 portable monitor and the polysomnogram. These data would determine the usefulness of the portable monitor for titration of the oral appliance as well as its use for confirmation of the effectiveness of the oral appliance in the management of the sleep apnea.

Another issue related to the use of the portable monitor by the nonphysician, in this case the dentist, is the cost. This applies to both the cost of the device, the cost for each test, and any related billing for the testing. The initial outlay for the portable monitor may be a concern. However, this has to be considered in relation to the potential savings in time that may be derived from being able to titrate the oral appliance more effectively and hence, decrease the number of follow-up visits for adjustment and modification, and may ultimately lead to more effective treatment outcomes. The situation as it relates to the cost for each test is directly related to the ability to charge or bill for the test. It is not advisable for the dentist to bill for any type of test that involves a diagnostic code for any type of sleep study or test. However, the cost to perform each test can adequately be absorbed into the fee for either the oral appliance or for the follow-up visit, depending on the fee structure or insurance contracted rates. The cost of each test needs to be considered when evaluating the various level 3 portable monitors that are available.

SUMMARY OF THE USE OF LEVEL 3 PORTABLE MONITORING RELATED TO ORAL APPLIANCE THERAPY

The following should be considered as it applies to the use of level 3 portable monitors related to the use of oral appliances:

1. The level 3 portable monitor is not to be used for initial screening or evaluation of patients with sleep-disordered breathing, particularly and solely by the dentist, who is advocating

the use of an oral appliance for the management of this condition.

2. The level 3 portable monitor can be used as an objective measurement device for the titration (adjustment and modification) of the oral appliance to achieve an optimum and effective outcome.

3. The portable monitor could be used at a future time to reevaluate the quality of sleep of the patient who is using an oral appliance when symptoms related to sleep-disordered breathing recur.

4. The portable monitor could be used to retest an oral appliance at various intervals in time to be certain that it is continuing to perform optimally. This might be done every 3 to 5 years.

5. The portable monitor can be used at the time when a replacement oral appliance is needed. It could be used to titrate the replacement oral appliance or to determine that it is functioning at the same level as the previous one. In this situation, the results of the testing would be compared with the subjective symptoms and their improvement.

6. The use of the portable monitor to evaluate the effect of the oral appliance ideally should also be able to test for sleep bruxism. A few devices currently may be able to do this but this is not part of the standard process.

These points are not meant to serve as guidelines but to begin to offer direction for the use of the level 3 portable monitor as it relates to both the dental sleep medicine practitioner and the use of oral appliances. Over time, clinical studies and continued development of level 3 portable monitors will support the development of more and better-defined guidelines and eventually will evolve into practice parameters that will better direct the use of the testing device. This will then enhance the effectiveness as well as the acceptance of oral appliances as a treatment of sleep apnea.

REFERENCES

1. Moses A. Protocol for primary treatment of snoring by dentists. Sleep Diagnosis and Therapy 2008; 3(6):21–2.

2. Levendowski DJ, Morgan T, Patrickus JE, et al. In-home evaluation of efficacy and titration of a mandibular advancement device for obstructive sleep apnea. Sleep Breath 2007;11(3):139–47.

3. Collop NA, McDowell W, Boehlecke B, et al. Clinical guidelines for the use of unattended portable monitors in the diagnosis of obstructive sleep apnea in adult patients. J Clin Sleep Med 2007; 3(7):737–47.

4. Bailey DR. Oral and nasal airway screening by the dentist. Sleep Med Clin 2010;5(1):1–8.

5. Collop NA. Home sleep testing – it is not about the test. Chest 2010;138(2):245.

6. Westbrook PR, Levendowski DJ, Cvetinovic M, et al. Description and validation of the apnea risk evaluation system – a novel method to diagnose sleep apnea-hypopnea in the home. Chest 2005;128(4): 2166–75.

7. Erman MK, Stewart D, Einhorn D, et al. Validation of the ApneaLink for screening of sleep apnea: a novel and simple single-channel recording device. J Clin Sleep Med 2007;3(4):387–92.

8. Chen H, Lowe AA, Bai Y, et al. Evaluation of a portable recording device (ApneaLink) for case selection of obstructive sleep apnea. Sleep breath 2009;13:213–9.

9. Epstein LJ, Kristo D, Strollo PJ, et al. Clinical guideline for the evaluation, management and long-term care of obstructive sleep apnea in adults. J Clin Sleep Med 2009;5(3):263–76.

10. Kushida CA, Morgentahler TI, Littner MR, et al. Practice parameters for the treatment of snoring and obstructive sleep apnea with oral appliances: an update for 1995. Sleep 2006;29(2):240–3.

11. ADSM Position Paper: Dental sleep medicine & portable monitoring. Report of the ADSM board of directors in dialogue. Dialogue 2005; issue 2. p. 10–2.

12. AADSM Treatment Protocol. Updated AADSM treatment protocol: oral appliance therapy for sleep disordered breathing. Dialogue 2009; issue 3. p 10.

13. Littner MR. Ambulatory testing for adult obstructive sleep apnea for the dentist. Sleep Med Clin 2010; 5(1):99–108.

14. Guimaraes KC, Drager LF, Genta PR, et al. Effects of oropharyngeal exercises on patients with moderate obstructive sleep apnea syndrome. Am J Respir Crit Care Med 2009;179:962–6.

15. McLornan P, Verrett R, Girvan T, et al. Evaluation of obstructive sleep apnea: patient's oral appliance titration protocols. Sleep Breath 2010;14:273–84 [abstract: P16].

Use of Portable Monitoring for Diagnosis and Follow-Up of Sleep-Disordered Breathing Treated With Upper Airway Surgery

Kavita Mundey, MD[a,b,*], Shilpa Guggali, MD[c],
B. Tucker Woodson, MD[d]

KEYWORDS

- Obstructive sleep apnea • Upper airway surgery
- Portable monitoring • Ambulatory sleep study

Obstructive sleep apnea (OSA) is a common condition that affects up to 24% of men and 9% of women.[1,2] When untreated, OSA increases risk of cardiovascular morbidity and mortality, motor vehicle accidents, metabolic abnormalities, and cognitive disturbances.[3–16] Treatment is associated with improvement in daytime somnolence, neurocognitive function, hypertension, and left ventricular function, and a decrease in health care costs.[17–22] Heightened awareness of effects of OSA on health has led to a burgeoning demand for diagnostic and therapeutic interventions. However, uncertainty and controversy surround many available options.

IDEAL TESTING FOR OSA: INDIVIDUALIZED APPLICATION OF AVAILABLE OPTIONS

The ideal test to confirm OSA is considered to be a technician-monitored in-laboratory polysomnogram.[23]

It identifies sleep stages, abnormal breathing events, limb movements, and selected electroencephalogram and electrocardiogram rhythm abnormalities. Despite its broad diagnostic potential, polysomnogram has evolved primarily into a diagnostic test for sleep apnea. It allows confirmation of disease, assessment of disease severity, and technician-supervised positive airway pressure (PAP) titration within a single night. However, it is also resource-intensive, expensive, and not readily available in all communities. Worldwide, the demand for polysomnogram testing is not matched by current resources.[24] Moderate to severe sleep apnea remain undiagnosed in 82% of men and 93% of women.[25] These statistics have helped fuel the debate over the use of alternative diagnostic methods, such as portable sleep monitoring (PM). Much of the debate has centered on technical issues, such as inability of PM to

Financial disclosure: Drs Mundey and Guggali have nothing to disclose. Dr Woodson has been a scientific consultant to Medtronic ENT, Inspire Medical, Aspire Medical, Resmed, Johnson & Johnson, and Siesta Medical and has received research support from Inspire Medical and royalties for a hyoid suspension device from Medtronic ENT.

a Clement J. Zablocki Veteran Affairs Medical Center, 5000 West National Avenue, Milwaukee, WI 53295, USA
b Division of Pulmonary, Critical Care and Sleep Medicine, Medical College of Wisconsin, 9200 West Wisconsin Avenue, Milwaukee, WI 53226, USA
c Department of Psychiatry and Behavioral Medicine, The Medical College of Wisconsin, 8701 Watertown Plank Road, Milwaukee, WI 53226, USA
d Department of Otolaryngology and Communication Sciences, Medical College of Wisconsin, 9200 West Wisconsin Avenue, Milwaukee, WI 53226, USA
* Corresponding author. Clement J. Zablocki Veteran Affairs Medical Center, 5000 West National Avenue, Milwaukee, WI 53295.
E-mail address: kmundey@mcw.edu

Sleep Med Clin 6 (2011) 341–347
doi:10.1016/j.jsmc.2011.05.006
1556-407X/11/$ – see front matter. Published by Elsevier Inc.

measure sleep time, sleep stages, accurate apnea-hypopnea index (AHI), or leg movements. Although factors that affect sleep study accuracy and reproducibility are not limited to PM monitoring, and may also apply to polysomnography, appropriate clinical assessment before therapy is a key issue, especially before more invasive surgical interventions.

The assessment and critical review of PM testing has often been performed when positive airway pressure (PAP) therapy is first-line therapy.[26] Before the advent of autotitrating PAP devices (APAP), few objective options existed for setting pressure requirements for patients. Although in-laboratory PAP titration studies are required for some patients, non–sleep laboratory titration of PAP using APAP devices is an effective and convenient alternative for many patients. Consequently, the need for routine polysomnography is increasingly questioned.

In patients undergoing surgery for OSA, however, this is not the case. Surgical therapies widely vary in their invasiveness and risk. High-quality data on the clinical effectiveness of many surgical procedures are lacking. Surgical procedures are widely accepted to have a variable and often poorly predictable effect on AHI, which has become the primary surrogate marker of sleep apnea disease severity. These differing clinical factors alter the dynamics of diagnostic testing and decision making in patients undergoing surgery for OSA. Because of the wide variability in both the application and interpretation of PM monitoring, it is difficult to argue for its routine use as a sole diagnostic method before major upper airway surgery. Current guidelines support using attended polysomnography and not PM for major upper airway reconstructive surgery.

However, depending on a variety of clinical situations, a need exists for differing types and levels of diagnostic testing in surgical sleep medicine. This argument is highlighted by the following cases. In case one, a healthy but overweight 22-year-old college student with complaints of snoring and daytime sleepiness but without hypertension or a regular bed partner is to undergo airway (nasal) surgery for deviated nasal septum. PM is negative for OSA. In case two, a patient has undergone PM testing for suspected sleep apnea and has a positive study with AHI of 48 events per hour after manual review. She is unable to tolerate continuous PAP. The questions raised in both cases are whether the patients now require in-laboratory attended polysomnography simply to receive the next therapeutic option (ie, potential surgical treatment), and whether the polysomnography (or for that matter a Multiple Sleep Latency Test [MSLT]) would change management at this point. Although clinicians have argued that polysomnography testing helps avoid suboptimal care, no actual patient data support this approach. A more appropriate argument is that suboptimal care is best addressed through proper training of medical and surgical sleep specialists rather than restricting use of effective diagnostic and treatment systems.

CURRENT GUIDELINES ON ROLE OF PORTABLE MONITORING

Few studies have assessed the clinical impact of PM on OSA treatment use and management. Consensus-based guidelines exist but fail to address unmet clinical needs.

The various types of available sleep monitoring systems are reviewed in **Table 1**. Attended polysomnography (type 1 study) is historically considered the ideal test; it confirms OSA and reveals other coexistent sleep disorders. In the proper setting (**Box 1**), PM represents an efficient method for diagnosing moderate and severe OSA.[26] The American Academy of Sleep Medicine (AASM) recommends the use of type 3 PM for diagnosis,

Table 1
AASM categories of sleep monitoring systems

Device	Parameters Measured
Type 1	Standard, in-laboratory, technician-attended, overnight PSG Minimum of seven channels, including EEG, EOG, chin EMG, EKG, oxygen saturation, airflow, respiratory effort
Type 2	Unattended PSG PM Minimum of seven channels, including EEG, EOG, chin EMG, EKG, oxygen saturation, airflow, respiratory effort
Type 3	Minimum of four channels, including ventilation or airflow (at least two channels of respiratory movement, or respiratory movement and airflow), heart rate, or EKG, and oxygen saturation
Type 4	One or two channels, typically including oxygen saturation or airflow

Abbreviations: EEG, electroencephalogram; EKG, electrocardiogram; EMG, electromyogram; EOG, electrooculogram; PM, portable sleep monitoring; PSG, polysomnogram.

Data from Collop NA, Anderson WM, Boehlecke B, et al. Clinical guidelines for the use of unattended portable monitors in the diagnosis of obstructive sleep apnea in adult patients. J Clin Sleep Med 2007;3:737–47.

Box 1
Necessary conditions for diagnosing moderate to severe OSA based on portable sleep systems[a]

1. A high pretest probability ideally to exceed 70% (ie, a high prevalence of obstructive sleep apnea/hypopnea syndrome; two or more of the following comorbid conditions: snoring, excessive daytime sleepiness, obesity, hypertension).
2. The availability of a type 1 study for patients with a strong clinical history and a negative or nondiagnostic PM.
3. The availability of treatment (currently PM can be used only when considering noninvasive treatment of OSA).
4. An experienced sleep practitioner capable of evaluating both the clinical and PM information (mandatory manual review of PM data).
5. The ability of type 3 PM devices to perform their identified function; capabilities and limitations of each device must be taken into account by the interpreter.
6. Result should be reported as positive (estimated AHI≥15) or negative (estimated AHI<15) for moderate to severe OSA rather than in terms of AHI for greatest accuracy of reported results.

[a] Based on AASM guidelines.
   Data from Collop NA, Anderson WM, Boehlecke B, et al. Clinical guidelines for the use of unattended portable monitors in the diagnosis of obstructive sleep apnea in adult patients. J Clin Sleep Med 2007;3:737–47.

whereas the Centers for Medicare & Medicaid Services (CMS) consider type 2 and type 3 PM systems acceptable. CMS also accepts type 4 systems measuring at least three channels.[26,27]

Guidelines have required manual confirmation of PM data for accuracy. No studies are available to guide use of PM for diagnosing sleep disorders other than OSA. Data on accuracy of PM are inadequate in patients with significant comorbid conditions (eg, severe pulmonary disease, neuromuscular disease, congestive heart failure), pediatric populations, and elderly populations (>65 years of age), and results should be interpreted with caution in these groups. For similar reasons, current guidelines restrict therapeutic options to nonsurgical treatments when PM is used to diagnose OSA.[26]

OPTIMAL TREATMENT FOR OSA: INDIVIDUALIZED APPLICATION OF AVAILABLE OPTIONS

Often the best outcomes of chronic disease management require more than a single intervention. For OSA, interventions may include[1] treating predisposing conditions (eg, obesity, hypothyroidism, nasal obstruction),[2] use of devices (eg, PAP, oral devices), and[3] surgery. PAP treatment has been accepted as the preferred treatment for OSA, showing an in-laboratory reduction of AHI to fewer than 5 events per hour.[28,29] In clinical populations, use of PAP for 4 hours per night for 5 to 7 nights per week is defined as "good compliance." However, this definition simply reflects the observation that most patients are unable to use continuous PAP regularly through the sleep period.[30] It is largely ignored that this pattern implies lack of treatment of OSA for approximately 50% of sleep time. Concurrently, many surgical options have been rejected because they do not consistently decrease AHI to fewer than 15 events per hour. Upper airway surgeries have not been shown to be inferior to PAP in improving clinical outcomes.[31] Additionally, up to 50% of adults are not compliant with PAP therapy.[32–36] For this large population, alternative treatment is required. Oral appliances, weight loss, positional therapies, bariatric surgery, and upper airway reconstructive surgeries are some of the currently available treatment options.

In the surgical management of OSA, treatment intent may be curative, salvage, or ancillary (Box 2). In a chronic disease, such as sleep apnea, "curative intent" is an inappropriate term because it may questionable whether a cure exists. Cure implies that disease is eliminated. Rarely, isolated anatomic abnormalities exist that, when corrected, are highly likely to eliminate OSA. A more appropriate term may be "definitive treatment." Definitive treatment reduces disease burden of symptoms and disease morbidity for an extended period without the need for other major therapies. The strategy for successful definitive treatment may be influenced by economic and medical costs of the disease and the risk/benefit ratio of the proposed therapy compared with alternative therapeutic options.

Salvage therapy treats patients after failure of first-line therapies. As a salvage treatment, the ideal outcome is definitive treatment. However,

Box 2
Goals of surgical treatment in patients with OSA

1. Curative: Correction of craniofacial structure with goal of eliminating OSA
2. Ancillary: Upper airway surgery not primarily targeted at eliminating OSA
3. Salvage: Second-line treatment after failure of first-line therapy

successful salvage treatment may be defined in relation to the cost of untreated disease without PAP therapies.

Finally, treatment intent may be ancillary. This intent is to combine the ancillary therapy with the primary or more conservative therapies to add to therapeutic benefit. The benefit from ancillary therapies, which are likely to be less invasive, is potentially and overwhelmingly the greatest of all the therapeutic options. Because the goal of ancillary treatment options is not definitive treatment of OSA, outcomes are virtually impossible to measure using the polysomnography measures and metrics.

UPPER AIRWAY SURGERY FOR OSA: POTENTIAL ROLE FOR PM

Airway obstruction in OSA occurs in complex anatomic structures of the supraglottic upper airway, including the nose, nasopharynx, oropharynx, and hypopharynx. To address these complex patterns of airway obstruction, various algorithms or "recipes" have been developed and advocated to treat sleep-disordered breathing, such as the two-phase Stanford treatment algorithm described by Riley and colleagues.[37] Other combinations of soft tissue procedures and isolated palatopharyngoplasty have been described. No direct comparative evidence supports one approach over others. Although, a wide variety of outcomes are reported for various procedures, often little information is provided on the nature of the population treated, making extrapolation to other patient groups difficult.

In expert hands, aggressive maxillomandibular advancement (MMA) has high success rates. No single algorithm for MMA exists, but most case series report a success rate of greater than 90% based on reduction of AHI to fewer than 10 events per hour.[38–41] Other sleep apnea surgeries, although not always curative for OSA, may improve clinical outcomes, such as symptoms, quality of life, cardiovascular events, and accident rates.[42–46]

Nasal surgery has the potential to treat multiple aspects of sleep-disordered breathing. Altering fixed upper airway resistance has marked impact on ventilation and sleep quality. Data suggest that outcomes associated with PAP, oral appliance therapy, and surgical treatment for OSA are improved and sleep quality is significantly affected.[42,43,45–48] Despite these effects and the undisputed contribution of nasal resistance to OSA, some have inappropriately criticized nasal treatments as ineffective based on traditional polysomnography outcomes.

Both the clinical indications and the effectiveness of nasal surgery must assess correct clinical outcomes. For most ancillary therapies, repeat objective testing will only confirm the continued presence of OSA. However, change in disease severity may occur that would alter management decisions in selected patients.

As described by Fujita and colleagues,[49] uvulopalatopharyngoplasty (UPPP) is a mucosal and tonsillar excisional procedure that has a dramatic effect on snoring but a limited effect on AHI in many patients. UPPP rarely cures the disease, and an overreliance on the procedure, inaccurate nomenclature, and incorrect description of outcomes have contributed to much of the controversy related to surgery for sleep apnea. Recent studies, however, confirm that adult subgroups exist who respond better to UPPP as an isolated procedure compared with other patient groups.[50] Furthermore, UPPP techniques continue to evolve. Several randomized clinical trials ignored by clinical reviews have shown a significant improvement in these techniques compared with initial descriptions.[51,52]

Techniques matter. Technical evolution to include lateral pharyngoplasty, expansion sphincterpharyngoplasty, the "Han UPPP," the extended uvulopalatal flap, and other advancement techniques promise lesser morbidity and improved effectiveness. Often surgical algorithms to reconstruct the upper airway are staged to maximize effectiveness and minimize morbidity. The use of clinical symptoms alone to assess residual disease severity is markedly limited. PM monitoring allows for interval testing of disease before proceeding with further stages of treatment. This testing during staged surgery is the surgical equivalent of PAP titration with medical therapy.

A wide variety of techniques have been described to alter other pharyngeal structures. Effectiveness of these is controversial and each has associated morbidity that must be balanced with outcomes. These techniques include limited surgical osteotomies of the anterior mandible, pharyngeal suspension using fascia, suture, or other novel implants. Hyoid suspension performed by pulling the hyoid forward to the mandible or to the more anteriorly situated thyroid cartilage has been described. The ideal candidates for many of these procedures have not been identified. Clinical decision making is based on anatomic and structural features determined through clinical examination, radiographic tools, or endoscopy. Because some procedures are more invasive than others and have greater risks and side effects, they are often offered to individuals with more severe disease. Sleep testing is not used for selection but contributes in assessing disease risk. This testing can also be used to assess outcomes after interval treatment and final treatment. PM monitoring is often ideal in these cases to allow repeated and frequent assessments to augment traditional level one testing.

Diagnosis of OSA may also be required in individuals who are undergoing upper airway surgery for conditions other than OSA. Patients with tonsillar hypertrophy, airway tumors, laryngeal or tracheal pathology, or acromegaly may all benefit from OSA testing. Symptom-based OSA screening criteria are often ignored or inadequate in many patients. The use of PM monitoring in appropriate individuals may provide a way to identify those at real risk of OSA-related adverse outcomes. In a small but not insignificant number of young adult patients with enlarged lymphoid tissue, surgical treatment may be curative for OSA. Furthermore, lymphoid tissue enlargement in older adults may not always be benign and should never be ignored, irrespective of sleep apnea treatment outcomes.

Current guidelines allow PM monitoring to be used during follow-up evaluation after surgery.[26] If the PM sleep study is negative in an asymptomatic patient, further intervention is not required. If the PM monitoring is positive for sleep apnea, further treatment is required, in the form of additional medical or surgical therapy. Conversely, a negative PM sleep study in symptomatic patients necessitates additional clinical evaluation, which may include repeat PM monitoring, a type 1 study, or additional testing, such as the MSLT, to look for other comorbid sleep disorders. One advantage of PM monitoring is the ability to perform multiple studies in a more natural environment.

SUMMARY

Treatment of OSA should be individualized based on patient preference and available resources. Patients must be aware of risks, benefits, and likely outcomes. Often patients will select procedures and algorithms that are perceived to have the lowest invasiveness and morbidity. Both PM sleep study and upper airway surgery have an undeniably important role. Currently, outcomes-based data are inadequate to guide optimal implementation of these modalities. The common-sense application of guidelines for use of PM in upper airway surgery involves a comprehensive clinical evaluation, patient counseling, and close follow-up after intervention. Prospective evaluation of outcomes would allow long-overdue evolution of the roles of these modalities.

REFERENCES

1. Young T, Palta M, Dempsey J, et al. The occurrence of sleep disorder breathing among middle age adults. N Engl J Med 1993;328:1230–5.
2. Duran J, Esnaola S, Rubio R, et al. Obstructive sleep apnea-hypopnea and related clinical features in a population-based sample of subjects aged 30 to 70 yr. Am J Respir Crit Care Med 2001;163(3): 685–9.
3. Peker Y, Hedner J, Kraiczi H, et al. Respiratory disturbance index: an independent predictor of mortality in coronary artery disease. Am J Respir Crit Care Med 2000;162:81–6.
4. Gami AS, Howard DE, Olson EJ, et al. Day-night pattern of sudden death in obstructive sleep apnea. N Engl J Med 2005;352:1206.
5. Young T, Peppard P, Palta M, et al. Population-based study of sleep-disordered breathing as a risk factor for hypertension. Arch Intern Med 1997;157(15): 1746–52.
6. Shahar E, Whitney CW, Redline S, et al. Sleep-disordered breathing and cardiovascular disease: cross-sectional results of the Sleep Heart Health Study. Am J Respir Crit Care Med 2001;163(1):19–25.
7. Peker Y, Kraiczi H, Hedner J, et al. An independent association between obstructive sleep apnoea and coronary artery disease. Eur Respir J 1999;14:179.
8. Baguet JP, Barone-Rochette G, Lévy P, et al. Left ventricular diastolic dysfunction is linked to severity of obstructive sleep apnea. Eur Respir J 2010;36: 1323–9.
9. Nieto JF, Young TB, Lind BK, et al. Association of SDB, sleep apnea and hypertension in a large community based study. JAMA 2000;283:1829–36.
10. Peppard PE, Young T, Palta M, et al. Prospective study of the association between sleep-disordered breathing and hypertension. N Engl J Med 2000; 342(19):1378–84.
11. Yaggi HK, Concato J, Kernan WN, et al. Obstructive sleep apnea as a risk factor for stroke and death. N Engl J Med 2005;353(19):2034–41.
12. Gruber A, Horwood F, Sithole J, et al. Obstructive sleep apnea is independently associated with the metabolic syndrome but not insulin resistance state. Cardiovasc Diabetol 2006;5:22.
13. Young T, Blustein J, Finn L, et al. Sleep-disordered breathing and motor vehicle accidents in a popular in a population-based sample of employed adults. Sleep 1997;20:608–13.
14. Howard ME, Desai AV, Grunstein RR, et al. Sleepiness, sleep-disordered breathing, and accident risk factors in commercial vehicle drivers. Am J Respir Crit Care Med 2004;170(9):1014–21.
15. Teran-Santos J, Jimenez-Gomez A, Cordero-Guevara J. The association between sleep apnea and the risk of traffic accidents. Cooperative Group

Burgos-Santander. N Engl J Med 1999;340(11): 847–51.

16. Kapur V, Bough DK, Sandblom RE, et al. The medical cost of undiagnosed sleep apnea. Sleep 1999;22:749.

17. Peker Y, Hedner J, Johansson A, et al. Reduced hospitalization with cardiovascular and pulmonary disease in obstructive sleep apnea patients on nasal CPAP treatment. Sleep 1997;20:645–53.

18. Bardwell WA, Ancoli-Israel S, Berry CC, et al. Neuropsychological effects of one-week continuous positive airway pressure treatment in patients with obstructive sleep apnea: a placebo-controlled study. Psychosom Med 2001;63:579.

19. Jenkinson C, Davies R, Mullins R, et al. Comparison of therapeutic and subtherapeutic nasal continuous positive airway pressure for obstructive sleep apnea: a randomized prospective parallel trial. Lancet 1999;353:2100–5.

20. Faccenda JF, Mackay TW, Boon NA, et al. Randomized placebo-controlled trial of continuous positive airway pressure on blood pressure in the sleep apnea-hypopnea syndrome. Am J Respir Crit Care Med 2001;163:344.

21. Aizpuru F, Pinto JA, Ayuela JM. Cardiac function after CPAP therapy in patients with chronic heart failure and sleep apnea: a multicenter study. Sleep Med 2008;9(6):660–6.

22. Bahammam A, Delaive K, Ronald J, et al. Health care utilization in males with obstructive sleep apnea syndrome two years after diagnosis and treatment. Sleep 1999;22:740–7.

23. Chesson AL, Ferber RA, Fry JM, et al. American sleep disorders association review: the indications for polysomnography and related procedures. Sleep 1997;20:423–87.

24. Flemons WW, Douglas NJ, Kuna ST, et al. Access to diagnosis and treatment of patients with suspected sleep apnea. Am J Respir Crit Care Med 2004; 169:668–72.

25. Young T, Evans L, Finn L, et al. Estimation of the clinically diagnosed proportion of sleep apnea syndrome in middle-aged men and women. Sleep 1997;20:705–6.

26. Collop NA, Anderson VM, Boehlecke B, et al; Portable Monitoring Task Force of the American Academy of Sleep Medicine. Clinical guidelines for the use of unattended portable monitors in the diagnosis of obstructive sleep apnea in adult patients. J Clin Sleep Med 2007;3(7):737–47.

27. Decision memo for continuous positive airway pressure (CPAP) therapy for obstructive sleep apnea (OSA) (CAG-00093R2). Available at: http://www.carolinasleepsociety.org/new/documents/cms_coverage_decision_memo_for_cpap.pdf. Accessed June 1, 2011.

28. Kushida CA, Littner MR, Hirshkowitz M, et al. Practice parameters for the use of continuous and bilevel positive airway pressure devices to treat adult patients with sleep-related breathing disorders. Sleep 2006;29:375–80.

29. Continuous positive airway pressure (CPAP) therapy for obstructive sleep apnea (OSA). Available at: https://www.cms.gov/transmittals/downloads/R150CIM.pdf. Accessed June 20, 2011.

30. Kribbs NB, Pack AL, Kline LR, et al. Objective measurement of patterns of nasal CPAP use by patients with obstructive sleep apnea. Am Rev Respir Dis 1993;147:887–95.

31. Powell N. Pro: upper airway surgery does have a major role in the treatment of obstructive sleep apnea "the tail end of the dog". J Clin Sleep Med 2005;1(3):236–40.

32. Meslier N, Lebrun T, Grillier-lanoir V, et al. A French survey of 3,225 patients treated with CPAP for obstructive sleep apnea: benefits, tolerance, compliance and quality of life. Eur Respir J 1998;12: 185–92.

33. Krieger J, Kurtz D, Petiau C, et al. Long term compliance with CPAP therapy in obstructive sleep apnea patients and in snorers. Sleep 1996;19:S136.

34. Grote L, Hedner J, Grunstein, et al. Therapy with nCPAP: incomplete elimination of sleep related breathing disorder. Eur Respir J 2000;16(5):921–7.

35. McArdle N, Devereux G, Heidarnejad H, et al. Long-term use of CPAP therapy for sleep apnea/hypopnea syndrome. Am J Respir Crit Care Med 1999; 159(4):):1108–14.

36. Rauscher H, Popp W, Wanke T, et al. Acceptance of CPAP therapy for sleep apnea. Chest 1991;100: 1019–23.

37. Riley RW, Powell NB, Guilleminault C, et al. Obstructive sleep apnea syndrome: a review of 306 consecutively treated surgical patients. Otolaryngol Head Neck Surg 1993;108(2):117–25.

38. Riley RW, Powell NB, Li KK, et al. Surgery and obstructive sleep apnea: long-term clinical outcomes. Otolaryngol Head Neck Surg 2000; 122(3):415–21.

39. Maurer Aurora RN, Casey KR, Kristo D, et al. Practice parameters for the surgical modifications of the upper airway for obstructive sleep apnea in adults. Sleep 2010;33(10):1408–13.

40. Conradt R, Hochban W, Heitmann J, et al. Sleep fragmentation and daytime vigilance in patients with OSA treated by surgical maxillomandibular advancement compared to CPAP therapy. J Sleep Res 1998;7(3):217–23.

41. Prinsell JR. Maxillomandibular advancement surgery in a site-specific treatment approach for obstructive sleep apnea in 50 consecutive patients. Chest 1999;116(6):1519–29.

42. Nakata S, Noda A, Yasuma F, et al. Effects of nasal surgery on sleep quality in obstructive sleep apnea syndrome with nasal obstruction. Am J Rhinol 2008;22(1):59–63.

43. Koutsourelakis I, Georgoulopoulos G, Perraki E, et al. Randomised trial of nasal surgery for fixed nasal obstruction in obstructive sleep apnoea. Eur Respir J 2008;31(1):110–7.

44. Fujita S. Midline laser glossectomy with linguoplasty: a treatment of sleep apnea syndrome. Op Tech Otolaryngol HNS 1991;2:127–31.

45. Li HY, Lin Y, Chen NH, et al. Improvement in quality of life after nasal surgery alone for patients with obstructive sleep apnea and nasal obstruction. Arch Otolaryngol Head Neck Surg 2008;134(4): 429–33.

46. Powell NB, Zonato AI, Weaver EM, et al. Radiofrequency treatment of turbinate hypertrophy in subjects using continuous positive airway pressure: a randomized, double-blind, placebo- controlled clinical pilot trial. Laryngoscope 2001;111:1783.

47. Sugiura T, Noda A, Nakata S, et al. Influence of nasal resistance on initial acceptance of continuous positive airway pressure in treatment for obstructive sleep apnea syndrome. Respiration 2007;74(1):56–60.

48. McLean HA, Urton AM, Driver HS, et al. Effects of treating severe nasal obstruction on the severity of obstructive sleep apnoea. Eur Respir J 2005;25: 521–7.

49. Fujita S, Conway W, Zorick F, et al. Surgical correction of anatomic abnormalities in obstructive sleep apnea syndrome: uvulopalatopharyngoplasty. Otolaryngol Head Neck Surg 1981;89:923–34.

50. Li HY, Wang PC, Lee LA, et al. Prediction of uvulopalatopharyngoplasty outcome: anatomy-based staging system versus severity-based staging system. Sleep 2006;29:1537–41.

51. Cahali MB, Formigoni GG, Gebrim EM, et al. Lateral pharyngoplasty versus uvulopalatopharyngoplasty: a clinical, polysomnographic and computed tomography measurement comparison. Sleep 2004;27(5): 942–50.

52. Pang KP, Woodson BT. Expansion sphincter pharyngoplasty: a new technique for the treatment of obstructive sleep apnea. Otolaryngol Head Neck Surg 2007;137(1):110–4.

Use of Portable Monitoring for the Diagnosis and Management of Sleep Disordered Breathing in Children: Highly Desirable, But Not Ready for Prime Time

Carol L. Rosen, MD[a,b,]*

KEYWORDS

- Sleep polysomnography • Child • Sleep apnea
- Obstructive sleep apnea • Diagnostic tests

Obstructive sleep apnea syndrome (OSAS) is a common condition of childhood with significant associated morbidity. Overnight attended recording and assessment of sleep and breathing by polysomnography (PSG) in a sleep laboratory have been traditional parts of the comprehensive evaluation of children who present signs and symptoms suggestive of OSAS. These studies require resources and facilities that are not always widely available. Simpler, more available, and less expensive alternatives have been sought. This article discusses the available alternatives to PSG for the evaluation of the child with suspected OSAS.

BACKGROUND OF GUIDELINES FOR PSG IN CHILDREN

In 1996, the American Thoracic Society published standards and indications for cardiopulmonary sleep studies in children.[1] PSG was recommended to differentiate benign snoring from pathologic snoring associated with OSAS. The document described various clinical scenarios where PSG was indicated and made specific recommendations for measures (respiratory and nonrespiratory), scoring, reporting, and conduct of the study. Although portable monitoring was not discussed, the document stated that if there were no clear-cut abnormalities on the respiratory portion of the PSG, then the study may be interpreted without performing complete staging. However, the writing group indicated that staging sleep and describing the sleep state dependence breathing were important parts of the documentation.

In 2002, the American Academy of Pediatrics (AAP) published a clinical practice guideline for the diagnosis and management of childhood OSAS accompanied by scientific review of the

This author has nothing to disclose.
[a] Division of Pediatric Pulmonary, Allergy and Immunology, and Sleep Medicine, University Hospitals-Case Medical Center, Case Western Reserve University School of Medicine, 11100 Euclid Avenue, RBC 793, Cleveland, OH 44106, USA
[b] Rainbow Babies and Children's Hospital, Pediatric Sleep Center, University Hospital Case Medical Center, 11100 Euclid Avenue, RBC 793, Cleveland, OH 44106, USA
* Division of Pediatric Pulmonary, Allergy and Immunology, and Sleep Medicine, University Hospitals-Case Medical Center, 11100 Euclid Avenue, RBC 793, Cleveland, OH 44106.
E-mail address: carol.rosen@case.edu

Sleep Med Clin 6 (2011) 349–353
doi:10.1016/j.jsmc.2011.05.009
1556-407X/11/$ – see front matter © 2011 Elsevier Inc. All rights reserved.

available literature.[2,3] This guideline contained the following recommendations for diagnostic evaluation:

> All children should be screened for snoring
> Complex high-risk patients should be referred to a specialist.
> Diagnostic evaluation is useful in discriminating between primary snoring and OSAS, the gold standard being PSG.

The documents reviewed various methods for OSAS diagnosis in childhood including history and physical examination, audiotaping or videotaping, pulse oximetry, abbreviated polysomnography, polysomnography during a daytime nap, and full overnight polysomnography. At that time, only a single center had published on home polysomnography in selected children, ages 2 to 12 years, using a specialized, noncommercial cardiorespiratory montage that included respiratory inductance plethysmography, oximetry, and oronasal airflow plus videotaping to estimate sleep/wake time.[4] The study compared the home-based findings with the in-laboratory recordings and reported close correlations. The AAP guideline concluded that while most studies had shown that abbreviated or screening techniques were helpful if positive, they had poor predictive value if negative. Thus, children with negative portable study results needed to undergo a more comprehensive in-laboratory evaluation. The cost efficacy of the screening techniques was unclear, and depended in part, on how may patients eventually required full polysomnography. Although overnight in-laboratory, attended PSG was recognized as the most reliable and objective test to assess presence and severity of OSAS,[2] data on the clinical utility of PSG were scant.

In 2011, the American Academy of Sleep Medicine (AASM) published new practice parameters for the respiratory indications for PSG in children[5] accompanied by a more detailed evidence-based executive summary.[6] In brief, the data indicated a strong clinical utility for PSG in children with suspected sleep disordered breathing (SDB) and obesity, evolving metabolic syndrome, neurologic, neurodevelopmental, or genetic disorders, and children with craniofacial syndromes. Specific consideration was given to the utility of PSG before adenotonsillectomy (AT) for confirmation of OSAS. The most relevant findings included: recognition that clinical history and examination are poor predictors of respiratory PSG findings; preoperative PSG is helping in predicting risk of perioperative complication; and preoperative PSG is often helpful in predicting persistence of OSAS in patients after AT. The authors concluded that PSG in children showed validity, reliability, and clinical utility. However, the gold standard for the diagnosis of SDB in children is not PSG alone, but rather the skillful integration of clinical and PSG findings by a knowledgeable sleep specialist. The document concluded that current evidence supports the clinical utility of PSG in the diagnosis and management of sleep-related breathing disorders in children. However, the accurate diagnosis in this population was best accomplished by integration of PSG findings with clinical evaluation. There was no discussion of portable monitoring in this document.

CURRENT THINKING ABOUT PORTABLE MONITORING IN CHILDREN

The role of portable monitoring in the evaluation and management of OSAS in adults is an area of active investigation,[7–9] with goals of increasing patient access and decreasing health care expenses. In children with suspected SDB, where access, services, and expertise are even more limited than in adults, home-based portable studies performed in the child's own bedroom would appear to be the ideal setting to evaluate sleep problems. To date, a clear role for ambulatory PSG in children has not been established. The following discussion summarizes new pediatric studies using portable monitoring technology in the evaluation of SDB since the original 2002 AAP guideline.

USING PORTABLE MONITORING TECHNOLOGY IN RESEARCH STUDIES

In the Cleveland Children's Sleep and Health study of the prevalence and health outcomes of SDB, a community-based sample of 907 children, ages 8 to 11 years, underwent overnight in-home cardiorespiratory recordings of respiratory effort (chest and abdomen), estimated airflow from the inductance bands, oximetry, electrocardiography, and body position.[10] On the evening of the study, a research assistant came to the family's home to place sensors on the child and instruct the parent about the device, which was picked up by a courier the following day. Technically acceptable studies were available in 94% of the samples.

In the Tucson's Children's Assessment of Sleep Apnea (TuCasa) study, a full in-home PSG with electroencephalogram (EEG) was performed by research staff who came to the family's home in the evening on the evening of the study. In the feasibility study, 157 of 162 (97%) studies were technically acceptable in children ages 5 to 12 years.[11]

The flow sensors were the most problematic in the TuCasa study, with thermistor and cannula having useable signal for only 59% and 52% of the total sleep time respectively. Of the sleep signals, the chin electromyogram (EMG) was poorest quality. Forty percent of the children said they slept somewhat worse that usual, and 6% reported much worse. The TuCasa study subsequently evaluated almost 500 children ages 6 to12 years using unattended evaluated full in-home PSG.[12]

Home PSG (standard sleep montage EEG, bilateral electro-oculogram [EOG], and chin EMG, leg EMG, oximetry, single piezo respiratory effort belt, and nasal oral thermistor) was used to evaluate sleep in 15 children with attention-deficit hyperactivity disorder (ADHD) (without psychiatric comorbidities, age range 7 to 11 years, not on medication) and in 23 healthy age-matched controls.[13] Sensors were applied at the home by an experienced PSG technologist, and the recording was supervised by that person. It is unclear from the publication whether the technologist remained in the home or supervised remotely. Compared with controls, the ADHD group had differences in sleep architecture, but did not have differences in SDB or periodic limb movements. Nasal pressure cannula was not used limited detection of hypopneas and SDB.

USING PORTABLE TECHNOLOGY FOR CLINICAL OSAS ASSESSMENTS IN OTHERWISE HEALTHY CHILDREN

In Canada, Kirk and colleagues[14] compared home oximetry monitoring with laboratory PSG in 58 children ages 4 to 14 with suspected OSAS. The PSG apnea–hypopnea index (AHI) agreed poorly with the portable monitor desaturation index. The sensitivity and specificity of the monitor for identification of moderate OSAS (defined as AHI >5) were 67% and 60%, respectively. The authors concluded that portable monitoring based on oximetry alone was not adequate for the identification of OSAS in otherwise healthy children.

Investigators in the Netherlands attempted to look at the clinical utility of a home-based, unattended cardiorespiratory monitor with a nasal cannula to diagnosis OSAS before adenotonsillectomy in symptomatic children.[15] Of 53 eligible children, only 24 participated in the study. The main reason for nonparticipation was refusal of caregivers (n = 16). Mean (standard deviation [SD]) age of participants was 4.2 (1.6) years. Technically acceptable recordings were obtained in 18 children (75%). Only 7 recordings (29%) were classified as successful. The poorest signal quality was obtained from the nasal cannula. The authors

concluded that the results of single-night unattended recordings at home fell short of their expectations.

Finally, investigators in Italy compared an abbreviated cardiorespiratory monitoring with PSG in 12 children (age range, 3 to 6 years) with suspected OSAS, but did not use the portable monitoring device unattended in a home environment.[16] The device included a nasal–oral thermistor, a snoring microphone, chest and abdominal respiratory effort sensors, a position sensor, a pulse oximeter, and single electrocardiogram (ECG) lead. The children underwent PSG and portable monitoring, both attended studies, on 2 different nights in a sleep laboratory, then compared the level of agreement between the two nights at two different respiratory disturbance index (RDI) index thresholds using the PSG data as the gold standard. In terms of correctly classifying the presence of OSAS, the level of agreement was low for RDI greater than 5 threshold and moderate for the RDI greater than 10 threshold. The portable device overestimated the number of central apneas and underestimated the obstructive hypopneas. The authors concluded that the device could not be recommended for common use in the clinical setting.

USING PORTABLE TECHNOLOGY FOR CLINICAL OSAS ASSESSMENTS IN MEDICAL COMORBIDITIES

Children with craniofacial disorders are at increased risk for developing OSAS. The feasibility of home cardiorespiratory monitoring using nasal airflow, oximetry, respiratory inductance plethysmography (RIP), and RIP-derived signal (X-flow) to estimate flow was evaluated in 129 children with craniosynostosis syndromes who underwent 200 different ambulatory PSGs[17] in the Netherlands. Compared with PSG, oximetry had a positive predictive value of 82% and a negative predictive value of 79% for the diagnosis of OSAS. Comparing the derived X-flow signal to the directly measured nasal pressure signal, 86% of the hypopneas and 55% of the obstructive apneas were correctly estimated, resulting in an underestimation of OSAS severity in 10% of patients. The investigators concluded that home cardiorespiratory monitoring was feasible; oximetry could be used as a rough estimate of severity, and X-flow can be helpful in diagnosing OSAS in the absence of nasal airflow.

Ambulatory physiologic monitoring that incorporated RIP technology to capture ventilation, pulse oximetry, single channels of ECG and EEG, and position, was used in a US study to assess the impact of aggressive pulmonary management strategies (noninvasive ventilation and airway clearance therapy) on sleep and breathing over a 3-month period in 8 patients ages 12 to 25 years with Duchenne muscular dystrophy.[18] Two patients withdrew during the study. In the remaining participants, respiratory rate decreased 10%, and sleep quality improved over the 3-month trial.

BARRIERS TO IMPLEMENTATION OF PORTABLE MONITORING IN CHILDREN

One important barrier to the implementation of portable monitoring has been the uncertainty about the respiratory indications and clinical utility of data from even in-laboratory, attended PSG in children. The need for PSG in otherwise healthy children and adolescents with suspected OSAS due to adenotonsillar hypertrophy remains controversial and has enormous cost implications. While the new practice parameters are a step forward in developing an evidence base and

---

Box 1
Barriers to implementation of unattended portable monitoring for clinical assessment of sleep-disordered breathing in children

Patient-related

Sensor loss (especially airflow-type)

Limited ability to cooperate to maintain sensor integrity (age or comorbidity-related)

Optimal target patient group

Family burden/acceptability of home studies

Requires parent/care-giver to stay up at night to monitor for sensor displacement

Accuracy and reliability of alternative ambulatory metrics for sleep-disordered breathing diagnosis and management decision

Thresholds for treatment or adverse health outcomes uncertain

Relationship between polysomnography and alternative portable monitoring metrics not established

Need of measuring sleep state, arousal, sleep fragmentation unknown

Strongest feasibility data from research settings

Limited data from clinical application-type studies were negative

Cost-effectiveness

Financial disincentive given uncertain reimbursement

---

building a consensus, debate remains. Many ear, nose, and throat (ENT) specialists do not routinely request PSG in children with suspected OSAS before AT.[19,20]

The American Academy of Otolaryngology–Head and Neck Surgery recently published a clinical practice guideline for tonsillectomy in children.[21] In that guideline, the clinical utility of PSG data was discussed. Although normative pediatric PSG data had been published,[22] and guidelines for performing and scoring PSGs in children were established,[23] there was no evidence-based consensus on a PSG-based cut-off value to indicate the need for treatment of OSAS. The authors concluded that any decision to recommend tonsillectomy should not be based solely on PSG findings, but should be based on clinical history, examination, and the likelihood that adenotonsillectomy will improve the SDB.

Other barriers to implementation of portable monitoring in children are listed in **Box 1**. Although feasibility of portable monitoring technology has been demonstrated in several pediatric groups, the majority of experience has been in a research setting. The most appropriate target population, the optimal limited channel montage, and validity of alternative SDB metrics where airflow is not directly measured have not been established. Cost-effectiveness has not been evaluated.

SUMMARY

Ideally, portable monitoring technology has the potential to increase patient access to sleep services, decrease the burden of sleep testing for young patients and their families, provide high-quality data, and reduce health care costs. Given the available data, the clinical applicability and role of portable monitoring in children have yet to be determined. The diagnosis of SDB in children is a difficult challenge even in an attended setting, especially in children less than 6 years of age or older children with limited ability to cooperate. Despite the standardization of PSG acquisition and scoring procedures in children and the development of evidence-based guidelines for PSG indications, the best SDB metrics to predict health outcomes and thresholds for recommending OSAS treatments are unknown. In this author's opinion, future investigations of the role of portable monitoring in children should focus on OSAS assessment of otherwise healthy adolescents and children with the more adult-like OSAS phenotype where the evidence for portable monitoring strategies is greater.

REFERENCES

1. American Thoracic Society. Standards and indications for cardiopulmonary sleep studies in children. Am J Respir Crit Care Med 1996;153:866.
2. Section on Pediatric Pulmonology, Subcommittee on Obstructive Sleep Apnea Syndrome. American Academy of Pediatrics. Clinical practice guideline: diagnosis and management of childhood obstructive sleep apnea syndrome. Pediatrics 2002;109:704.
3. Schechter MS. Technical report: diagnosis and management of childhood obstructive sleep apnea syndrome. Pediatrics 2002;109:e69.
4. Jacob SV, Morielli A, Mograss MA, et al. Home testing for pediatric obstructive sleep apnea syndrome secondary to adenotonsillar hypertrophy. Pediatr Pulmonol 1995;20:241.
5. Aurora RN, Zak RS, Karippot A, et al. Practice parameters for the respiratory indications for polysomnography in children. Sleep 2011;34:379.
6. Wise MS, Nichols CD, Grigg-Damberger MM, et al. Executive summary of respiratory indications for polysomnography in children: an evidence-based review. Sleep 2011;34:389.
7. Collop NA. Home sleep testing: it is not about the test. Chest 2010;138:245.
8. Collop NA. Portable monitoring for diagnosing obstructive sleep apnea: not yet ready for primetime. Chest 2004;125:809.
9. Collop NA, Anderson WM, Boehlecke B, et al. Clinical guidelines for the use of unattended portable monitors in the diagnosis of obstructive sleep apnea in adult patients. Portable Monitoring Task Force of the American Academy of Sleep Medicine. J Clin Sleep Med 2007;3:737.
10. Rosen CL, Larkin EK, Kirchner HL, et al. Prevalence and risk factors for sleep-disordered breathing in 8- to 11-year-old children: association with race and prematurity. J Pediatr 2003;142:383.
11. Goodwin JL, Enright PL, Kaemingk KL, et al. Feasibility of using unattended polysomnography in children for research—report of the Tucson Children's Assessment of Sleep Apnea study (TuCASA). Sleep 2001;24:937.
12. Goodwin JL, Silva GE, Kaemingk KL, et al. Comparison between reported and recorded total sleep time and sleep latency in 6- to 11-year-old children: the Tucson Children's Assessment of Sleep Apnea Study (TuCASA). Sleep Breath 2007;11:85.
13. Gruber R, Xi T, Frenette S, et al. Sleep disturbances in prepubertal children with attention deficit hyperactivity disorder: a home polysomnography study. Sleep 2009;32:343.
14. Kirk VG, Bohn SG, Flemons WW, et al. Comparison of home oximetry monitoring with laboratory polysomnography in children. Chest 2003;124:1702.
15. Poels PJ, Schilder AG, van den Berg S, et al. Evaluation of a new device for home cardiorespiratory recording in children. Arch Otolaryngol Head Neck Surg 2003;129:1281.
16. Zucconi M, Calori G, Castronovo V, et al. Respiratory monitoring by means of an unattended device in children with suspected uncomplicated obstructive sleep apnea: a validation study. Chest 2003;124:602.
17. Bannink N, Mathijssen IM, Joosten KF. Use of ambulatory polysomnography in children with syndromic craniosynostosis. J Craniofac Surg 2010;21:1365.
18. Landon C. Novel methods of ambulatory physiologic monitoring in patients with neuromuscular disease. Pediatrics 2009;123(Suppl 4):S250.
19. Mitchell RB, Pereira KD, Friedman NR. Sleep-disordered breathing in children: survey of current practice. Laryngoscope 2006;116:956.
20. Weatherly RA, Mai EF, Ruzicka DL, et al. Identification and evaluation of obstructive sleep apnea prior to adenotonsillectomy in children: a survey of practice patterns. Sleep Med 2003;4:297.
21. Baugh RF, Archer SM, Mitchell RB, et al. Clinical practice guideline: tonsillectomy in children. Otolaryngol Head Neck Surg 2011;144:S1.
22. Beck SE, Marcus CL. Pediatric polysomnography. Sleep Med Clin 2009;4:393.
23. Iber C, Ancoli-Israel S, Chesson A, et al. The AASM manual for scoring of sleep and associated events: rules, terminology and technical specification. 1st edition. Westchester (IL): American Academy of Sleep Medicine; 2007.

Portable Monitoring: Practical Aspects and Case Examples

Parina Shah, MD[a],*, Indira Gurubhagavatula, MD, MPH[a,b]

KEYWORDS

- Portable monitoring • Obstructive sleep apnea
- Positive airway pressure • Polysomnography
- Home sleep testing • Unattended sleep testing

Obstructive sleep apnea (OSA) is a medical condition that is strongly associated with obesity. The prevalence of OSA in the general population in 1993 was estimated to be 2% to 4%.[1] However, with the rising worldwide incidence of obesity, the percentage of patients with OSA is likely to be much higher. Most cases remain undiagnosed. Increased awareness of sleep apnea by primary care physicians and specialists has led to an increasing number of requests for sleep studies. The high prevalence of OSA, high expense of in-laboratory sleep studies, the current economic environment, and the rapid pace of technological advancement have all contributed toward the increased use of portable sleep monitoring for the diagnosis of OSA.

In March 2009, the Centers for Medicare and Medicaid Services (CMS) approved coverage for positive airway pressure (PAP) therapy for patients diagnosed with OSA using portable monitoring.[2,3] The authors expect that private insurance carriers are likely to follow suit, with hopes of reducing overall cost because the cost of an unattended sleep study performed in patients' homes is likely to be lower than comprehensive monitoring in the laboratory with a technician present. Comparative data regarding overall health care costs of OSA management using portable management versus pathways that require in-laboratory testing and PAP titration is limited. Nevertheless, the use of portable testing is likely to increase because

of the ease of application and because of the relative inaccessibility of in-laboratory testing.

This article reviews important aspects of portable sleep monitoring and provides clinical examples to aid the practitioner in the application of this rapidly evolving technology.

TYPES OF STUDIES

In 1994, the American Academy of Sleep Medicine (AASM) offered a classification system for the 4 types of monitors used for the diagnosis of sleep apnea.[4] A type 1 study is a standard in-laboratory polysomnography that is performed with a sleep technician in attendance. The distinct benefit of a standard polysomnogram is that an experienced technician is present to correct faulty signals in real time, increasing the likelihood of yielding an acceptable recording, and also to offer prompt continuous positive airway pressure (CPAP) treatment, if needed.[4] Because all sleep variables are recorded in this study, including electroencephalogram (EEG), electro-oculogram (EOG), and electromyogram (EMG), one can determine sleep staging, arousal index, and the presence of limb movements. This information allows for the diagnosis of positional and rapid eye movement (REM) sleep-related disorders, parasomnias, and disorders other than sleep apnea, such as periodic limb movement disorder.

[a] Division of Sleep Medicine, University of Pennsylvania, 3624 Market Street, Philadelphia, PA 19104, USA
[b] Pulmonary, Critical Care, and Sleep Section, Philadelphia VA Medical Center, Sleep Center, 3900 Woodland Avenue, Philadelphia, PA 19104, USA
* Corresponding author. University of Pennsylvania, 3624 Market Street, Suite 205, Philadelphia, PA 19104.
E-mail address: Parina.Shah@uphs.upenn.edu

Sleep Med Clin 6 (2011) 355–366
doi:10.1016/j.jsmc.2011.05.007
1556-407X/11/$ – see front matter. Published by Elsevier Inc.

Type 2, 3, and 4 sleep studies are portable, meaning they can be done outside of the laboratory. They do not require the presence of a technician, so neither the option of correcting faulty signals in real time, nor the prompt administration of treatment are available. A type 2 study is a portable polysomnography that includes the comprehensive signal montage used for the type 1 in-laboratory study, but without the presence of a technician, and can be performed at locations outside of the sleep laboratory, including patients' homes. As with a type 1 study, type 2 studies also record continuous EEG, allowing for the quantification of arousals, the staging of sleep, and the diagnosis of disorders other than sleep-disordered breathing. Although type 2 studies should theoretically be similar to in-laboratory studies in their ability to calculate accurate apnea-hypopnea index (AHI), sensitivity and specificity data is insufficient.[5] Type 3 and 4 studies typically do not include EEG monitoring.

A type 4 study is a continuous single- or dual-bioparameter recording that commonly records both the oxyhemoglobin saturation and the heart rate. Practice parameters for the use of portable monitoring, developed jointly in 2003 by the AASM, the American Thoracic Society, and the American College of Chest Physicians recommended that a type 4 study should not be used to diagnose sleep apnea or confirm an AHI greater than 15 because of insufficient evidence of such use.[5] In the outpatient setting, it may help to determine the need for additional home oxygen therapy in patients with OSA, overlap syndrome, or obesity hypoventilation syndrome (OHS). A type 4 study may have a greater diagnostic yield in patients with comorbidities, such as chronic obstructive pulmonary disease (COPD) and OHS, or those with lower functional residual capacity (eg, older age, abdominal obesity) who are more likely to demonstrate oxyhemoglobin desaturation.[6] It can also serve as a crude measurement of persistent apneas despite CPAP therapy, although many CPAP devices also offer treatment variables, including their estimation of residual apneas. Type 4 studies may be applied in inpatient settings where the presence of other electrical monitoring devices can interfere with high-quality signal acquisition that is required if more extended sleep-monitoring devices are to be used. Type 4 studies may signal a need for inpatient CPAP treatment in patients who are suspected to have the diagnosis, and may serve as crude markers of treatment success. However, they will not detect sleep-disordered breathing events that result in arousals, without oxyhemoglobin desaturation, such as some hypopneas or respiratory effort-related arousals (RERAs). Type 4 studies typically do not allow distinction between central and obstrucitve sleep apnea.

In the remainder of this discussion, the authors focus on type 3 studies, the type most commonly referenced when the term portable sleep apnea testing is used. According to AASM practice standards, a type 3 monitor must assess a minimum of 4 parameters. Of these, 2 must be respiratory parameters and the remaining 2 signals must measure heart rate/electrocardiogram (ECG) and oxyhemoglobin saturation. Respiratory parameters include movement (chest or abdomen) and airflow. A type 3 study typically does not measure EEG, EMG, and EOG. Although this type of study does not require the presence of a technician, if the situation requires it, a technician may remain in attendance to ensure proper signal acquisition and quality.

GENERAL ISSUES RELATED TO PORTABLE MONITORING AND AASM CLASSIFICATION

Portable monitors generally involve the use of nasal cannulas to record nasal air flow, abdominal and chest belts to record respiratory effort, and pulse oximetry to record heart rate and oxyhemoglobin saturation. The AASM recommends that ideally, portable monitors should use both an oronasal thermal sensor and a nasal pressure transducer to detect apneas,[7] but not all portable monitors offer these testing modalities. For instance, the examples provided in this article are derived from a portable monitoring system that only uses a nasal pressure transducer to detect respiratory events. Portable monitors can be rather heterogeneous. Because there are no standardized rules for data acquisition, signal types and sampling frequency vary widely between monitors, so data from one monitor may not be comparable to data from another. Some type 3 monitors may even offer 1 or 2 EEG channels. Another monitor has used changes in peripheral arterial tone as a marker of arousal activity, without direct EEG monitoring,[8] and, therefore, may not easily fall into one of the classes delineated by the AASM.

INDICATIONS FOR HOME PORTABLE MONITORING

In 2007, the AASM published clinical guidelines for the use of unattended portable monitors. An unattended portable study should only be performed in the setting of a comprehensive clinical evaluation by a board-certified sleep medicine specialist.[7] Its use should be limited to patients who have a high pretest probability of moderate to severe OSA.

Patients in whom other sleep disorders are being considered, including restless legs syndrome, nocturnal seizures, central sleep apnea, and REM sleep behavior disorder, require an in-laboratory study because the EEG and limb EMG are important components in determining the correct diagnosis.[7] The AASM does not list the use of supplemental oxygen as a contraindication for the use of portable monitoring.[7] Several studies that were used to validate portable monitors, however, specifically excluded those wearing supplemental oxygen.[7] Therefore, data regarding diagnostic efficacy in this particular group is sparser, and the authors think that portable monitors should be applied with caution in this group. Supplemental oxygen may decrease the likelihood of significant oxyhemoglobin desaturation occuring in association with respiratory events. The presence of EEG may allow greater scoring of hypopneas associated with arousal and therefore, obtain a more accurate estimate of apnea severity. According to AASM clinical guidelines, portable monitoring should not be used in patients with conditions that may degrade accuracy, including neuromuscular disease, severe pulmonary disease, or congestive heart failure.[7] These conditions may alter the accuracy of portable monitoring because of tremor, low baseline oxyhemoglobin saturations, or the presence of central apnea.

THE POTENTIAL FOR MISSED CASES WITH TYPE 3 PORTABLE MONITORS

Because type 3 studies typically do not include EEG monitoring, hypopneas that are clinically significant and lead to arousals (but without desaturation) and contribute to daytime sleepiness could potentially be missed. Similarly, RERAs, which can contribute to daytime sleepiness,[4] can be missed. In addition, total sleep time cannot be measured, so the denominator of the AHI is not actual sleep time, but a surrogate marker of sleep time. Some devices use test time to approximate sleep time, whereas others[9] incorporate activity monitors to differentiate between periods when patients are awake or asleep. Missed RERAs, hypopneas, or overestimation of sleep time may lead to an underestimation of the overall AHI and false negatives. Patients who may otherwise benefit from treatment may not receive it. Such patients include those who are less likely to experience oxyhemoglobin desaturation, such as populations that develop apnea at a younger age or lower body mass index (BMI) values.[10,11] For this reason, if the portable study is negative, a confirmatory in-laboratory, full sleep study is recommended by the AASM.[7]

IDEAL PATIENTS

In addition to meeting the previously mentioned indications for a portable sleep study, patients must exhibit sufficient cognitive skill and manual dexterity to assemble the study at home, or have a friend or family member who is able to complete the assembly of the device. Patients with certain medical conditions may, therefore, not be appropriate candidates for portable testing. On the other hand, patients whose typical sleep schedules do not coincide with the typical time of operation of a sleep laboratory, such as those with circadian sleep disorders, night-shift workers, and frequent travelers, may find home monitoring to be more suitable because they can wear the device during their typical sleep period in a location that is convenient for them.

PATIENT EDUCATION

Patient education for self-assembly of the device is requisite if the monitor is to be used in an unattended setting. An experienced technician or respiratory therapist could be trained to provide this service. Some institutions provide patient education through a teaching video. The portable device is often preprogrammed to begin recording at a set date and time when patients must perform the study. In patients with advanced or delayed phase syndromes and those who are shift workers, the study start time should be programmed at the patients' typical time of sleep. Patients are also provided instruction on how to apply the chest/abdominal belts and nasal thermistor and how to connect these to a data recorder. Some monitors require clothing between the patient and the device. Patients must have a sense of the appropriate tightness of the belts needed to record a rise or fall in the chest/abdomen. Patients must also be instructed to affix the airflow channel and pulse oximetry device in a way that minimizes the chance of dislodgement.

SCORING

Available data suggest that manual scoring may be superior to the automatic scoring offered by some monitors.[12] These internal scoring algorithms tend to be proprietary, require specific software, and are neither standardized nor transparent. The AASM recommends that once the study has been completed, raw data should be scored by a qualified and experienced sleep technologist. Current published AASM standards for scoring should be used to score respiratory events.[7] A hypopnea is defined by a drop in the nasal pressure signal amplitude by 30% or greater for at least 10 seconds and 90% of the event's duration. The respiratory event should be associated with a 4% or greater reduction in oxyhemoglobin saturation from the pre-event baseline.[13] **Fig. 1** demonstrates hypopneas on a portable study reading. One can see a reduction, not a complete cessation, of nasal airflow with associated oxyhemoglobin desaturations of 5 percentage points (top row) and increases in heart rate (bottom row) likely corresponding to posthypopnea arousals. **Fig. 2** demonstrates an example of an apnea, which is defined as a drop in peak airflow sensor excursion by 90% or greater than that of the baseline for 90% or greater than the duration of the event (which must be at least 10 seconds).[13] Importantly, the presence of a continued inspiratory effort, as demonstrated by the thoracic and abdominal excursion, indicates the apnea is an obstructive rather than central event. Since oral airflow may not be monitored with most portable devices, reductions due to mouth breathing may be incorrectly scored as hypopneas. Scoring algorithms may overlook nuances in the study that provide important clinical information. For example, **Fig. 3** demonstrates a postsigh apnea, also known as a Hering-Breuer inflation reflex. After a large inhaled breath, pulmonary stretch receptors in the airway smooth muscle cells send inhibitory signals through the vagus nerve to the respiratory control center in the brainstem. Inspiration is inhibited to prevent excessive stretching of the lung. A central apnea, which is a cessation in airflow without chest or abdominal effort, ensues. These apneas are considered part of a normal physiologic response. An automated program may score this as a central apneic event; however, a trained and experienced sleep

provider may choose to not mark this as a pathologic event.

Fig. 4 shows 2 central apneas. The first apnea occurs after a large inhalation or sigh. However, because this event is accompanied by relative bradycardia and followed by a large desaturation, it may be considered pathologic. Alternatively, the bradycardia may correspond to vagal inhibitory signals initiated by a sigh. The desaturation may have likely led to an arousal from sleep, which cannot be ascertained because of the absence of EEG monitoring. However, the purported arousal may have triggered the next sleep-onset central apnea, which occurs without a large preceding inhalation. Full EEG monitoring would have helped determine whether these events were a response to a sigh or an arousal. Central apneas can occur not only in the setting of sleep onset but also congestive heart failure, central nervous system disease, and initiation of CPAP or bilevel PAP therapy. Central apnea associated with PAP treatment may improve over time. Knowledge of the clinical information may assist the physician in gauging whether the central apnea is likely to be physiologic or pathologic. For these reasons, the sleep study should be read by an experienced sleep specialist who is knowledgeable about how to use clinical information and is aware of the limitations of this testing modality.

STRENGTHS OF PORTABLE MONITORING

One major advantage of the portable sleep study is that it can be conducted in patients' homes. A more representative night of sleep in terms of quality, quantity, and position is likely to be

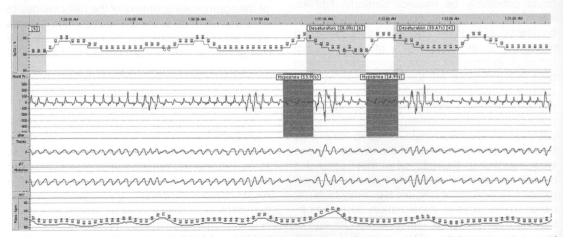

Fig. 1. An example of hypopneas from a type 3 recording. From top to bottom: oxyhemoglobin saturation, nasal airflow, thoracic movement, abdominal movement, and heart rate. This particular portable monitor only uses a nasal pressure transducer but does not use an oral thermistor. The AASM recommends that, ideally, portable monitors should use both types of channels.

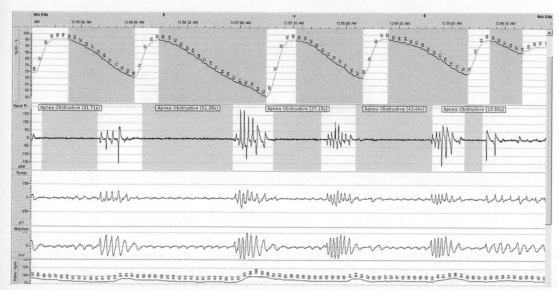

Fig. 2. An example of several obstructive apneas from a type 3 recording. This figure demonstrates (from *top* to *bottom*) oxyhemoglobin desaturation, nasal airflow, thoracic excursions, abdominal excursions, and heart rate. There is complete cessation of airflow without loss of respiratory effort, which is consistent with an obstructive event. Wide thoracic and abdominal excursions are present in association with resumption of airflow.

captured on the study because other factors that may interfere with sleep in the laboratory environment are not present. Such factors include the patients' perception of comfort of the bed, unfamiliarity of the surroundings, and discomfort caused by EEG lead placement. For these reasons, portable testing may uncover clandestine sleep apnea or REM-related sleep apnea that may be missed in an in-laboratory study.

Fig. 5 is a hypnogram that shows probable REM-related sleep apnea. Periodic oxyhemoglobin desaturations (second row) occur in conjunction with hypopnelc (third row) and apneic (fourth row) events, as well as increases in heart rate (fifth row). These events are not related to body position, which is indicated in the top row. The rise in heart rate (fifth row) clustered around these respiratory events suggests the presence

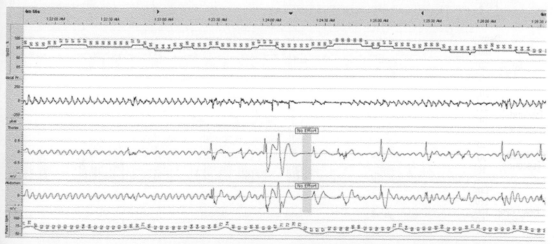

Fig. 3. Postsigh central apnea or Hering-Breuer inflation reflex from a type-3 recording. This event occurs after a large inhaled breath. Pulmonary stretch receptors in airway smooth muscle send inhibitory signals through the vagus nerve to the respiratory control center of the brainstem. As a result, inspiration is inhibited and a central apnea ensues.

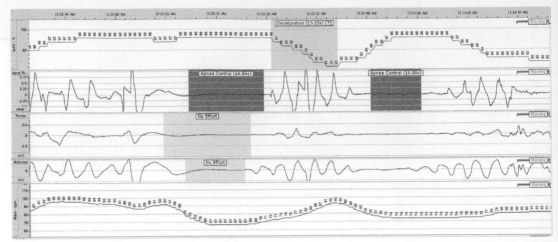

Fig. 4. Two central apneas from a type 3 recording. The first apnea occurs after a large inhalation (sigh); relative bradycardia accompanies the event and a large desaturation follows the event, so it may be considered pathologic. Alternatively, the bradycardia may correspond to vagal inhibitory signals from pulmonary stretch receptors. The second central apnea occurs without a large inhalation, but may have followed an arousal that terminated the first central apnea. Central apneas can occur in the setting of congestive heart failure, central nervous system disease, with initiation of CPAP/BPAP therapy, or with sleep onset.

of associated arousals. If patients are unable to achieve REM sleep (which may occur for some patients in the laboratory setting), he or she may have a negative study. Furthermore, the increased amount of REM sleep on this study is more likely to yield a higher AHI as compared to a study with minimal REM sleep. On the other hand, this study does not capture supine REM sleep, the condition under which sleep apnea is likely to be most severe. Technologists attending a sleep study can intervene during a recording to ensure that patients remain sleeping in the supine position, to increase diagnostic yield. The home portable sleep study may underestimate AHI because

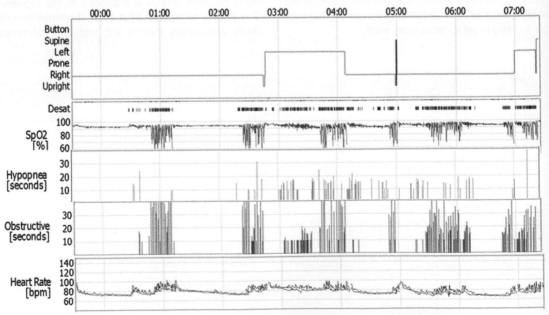

Fig. 5. REM-related sleep apnea from a type 3 recording. Intermittent oxyhemoglobin desaturation occurs with corresponding hypopneas and obstructive apneas in a repetitive pattern throughout the night, which is illustrative of REM-related sleep apnea. There is a corresponding increase in heart rate during these events, as would be seen during the termination of apneic events and the occurrence of arousals.

correction of body position would not be feasible, and more sleep may be observed in nonsupine positions, which may offer relative protection from apnea in a subgroup of patients.[14] One could argue, however, that if a patient does not habitually sleep on his or her back, demonstration of supine REM sleep may be less relevant.

Fig. 6 demonstrates an example of positional sleep apnea from a type 3 recording. Obstructive events with minor oxyhemoglobin desaturation are seen when the patient is in supine sleep. Alternatively, this hypnogram could represent severe apnea that occurs during supine REM sleep. Because a portable sleep study does not provide EEG data and sleep staging, this differentiation cannot be made. In an in-laboratory study, a technologist in attendance can ensure that greater amount of supine sleep is observed. Therefore, in this particular case, the AHI may have been higher. However, the AHI derived from this portable study may be more representative of the patient's typical nightly experience in his usual sleeping environment. Apnea was not observed during supine periods at the beginning of the study from about 23:00 to just after midnight. It is possible that the patient had not yet fallen asleep during that time, or that an additional condition, such as REM sleep, was not present at that time. The frequent changes in body position suggest that the patient was likely awake during this period.

Although AASM clinical guidelines recommend portable monitoring should not be used in patients with congestive heart failure, central apnea can be seen on portable studies (see **Figs. 3** and **4**). While no large studies have been performed to determine the sensitivity and specificity of portable monitors to detect central sleep apnea, a European study of 75 patients with congestive heart failure yielded a sensitivity and specificity of 100% when compared with in-laboratory polysomnography.[15] Many of these patients have both OSA and central sleep apnea, the former often being a cause or factor contributing to congestive heart failure and the latter being a manifestation of it. **Fig. 7** shows an example of the Cheyne-Stokes breathing pattern in a patient with congestive heart failure from a type 3 recording. The 2007 AASM manual for scoring defines Cheyne-Stokes breathing as at least 3 consecutive cycles of cyclic crescendo and decrescendo patterned breathing that occurs for at least 10 consecutive minutes or occurs in conjunction with at least 5 central apneas or hypopneas per hour of sleep.[13] The cycle length is typically in the range of 60 seconds.[13] In this particular patient, this pattern of breathing continued for several minutes.

These patients should be brought to the laboratory to undergo titration with CPAP, and if not effective, with either bilevel PAP, possibly with a timed mode, or adaptive or auto servo-ventilation, a more sophisticated means of PAP treatment that treats both OSA and central apnea.[16] This population is very important and relevant and would gain greater access to sleep testing through the use of portable monitoring. Testing is particularly important in patients with congestive heart failure because treatment of their underlying apnea may offer cardiovascular benefit, and the presence of central apnea may be an indicator of suboptimal medical therapy of the heart failure.

Type 3 portable testing eliminates the expense and inconvenience of a sleep technician traveling to the patients' location, as in a type 2 study. AASM clinical guidelines by the portable monitoring task force state that portable monitoring

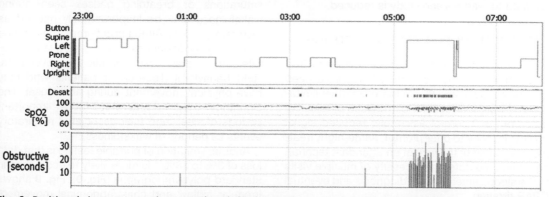

Fig. 6. Positional sleep apnea. The second and third rows show a cluster of oxyhemoglobin desaturations and obstructive events when the patient is in the supine position, seen in the top row. Apnea was not observed during supine periods at the beginning of the study from about 23:00 to just after midnight. It is possible that the patient had not yet fallen asleep during that time. The frequent changes in body position suggest that the patient was probably awake during this period.

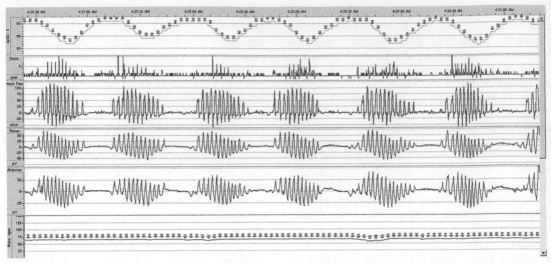

Fig. 7. Cheyne-Stokes breathing pattern from a type 3 recording. This image is a snapshot of an unattended sleep study in a 65-year-old man with a history of congestive heart failure. Phasic decreases in oxyhemoglobin saturation, nasal airflow, and chest and abdominal excursions represent central sleep apneas. The periodic nature of these events is consistent with Cheyne-Stokes respiration, which can be seen in patients with congestive heart failure. The cycle length is typically in the range of 60 seconds. In this particular patient, this pattern of breathing continued for several minutes. This patient was referred for bilevel PAP titration.

may be a reasonable option in patients "for whom in-laboratory polysomnogram (PSG) is not possible by virtue of immobility, safety, or critical illness.[7]" This type is especially an advantage in patients with anxiety, posttraumatic stress disorder, morbid obesity, chronic back pain, neuromuscular disease, stroke, physical handicap, or mental retardation.

Although portable monitoring is generally done in the home, it can also be used in other settings, such as nursing homes, rehabilitation facilities, and inpatient facilities.[6] Because of the absence of EEG and EMG data, the duration of time required to read a sleep study is reduced.

LIMITATIONS OF PORTABLE MONITORING

Portable home monitoring carries limitations. The most obvious one is the inability to record a sleep EEG (see **Figs. 5** and **6**), but there are other limitations as well, such as data loss caused by a lack of assembly or incorrect assembly; reduced signal quality; inability to offer prompt, same-night treatment because of the lack of an attendant technologist; and the potential necessity of multiple visits to the sleep center for OSA diagnosis and eventual CPAP titration.

As previously mentioned, overestimated sleep time and missed RERAs can lead to underestimation of actual AHI. However, some newer portable monitors have incorporated actigraphy as a marker

of sleep and wakefulness as a mechanism to determine the total sleep time.[9] **Fig. 8** demonstrates how actigraphy may be useful. The respiratory events occur throughout the night except for the first few hours of the night, when activity is noted to be high, indicating that the patient is likely awake. This point is further supported by frequent changes in body position, as seen in the top row, which occur at the same time. In this case, based on actigraphy, the total sleep time is less than the total recording time. Therefore, the calculated AHI would be higher than if the study did not incorporate actigraphy. Furthermore, oxyhemoglobin desaturations or breathing pauses seen during wakefulness may be inappropriately marked as respiratory events. Although actigraphy has proven useful in some instances, it may yield a less accurate AHI in patients with periodic leg movements, REM behavioral disorder, or patients who may have physical movement during an arousal. The algorithm may misinterpret these important periods of sleep and their associated respiratory events as periods of wakefulness.

Another limitation of portable testing is that data loss of 3% to 18%[17] is more likely to occur than in standard polysomnography (**Fig. 9**). **Fig. 9** shows irregular airflow and chest/abdominal movement waveforms indicating movement, which is confirmed by actigraphy. This movement leads to the transient loss of data, likely from dislodgement of the pulse oximeter. Such data loss may

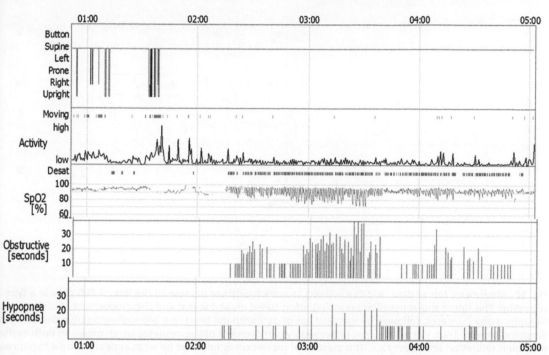

Fig. 8. Nocturnal actigraphy from a type 3 recording. This figure illustrates actigraphy (*second row*). The respiratory events occur throughout the night, except for the first few hours of the night, when activity is noted to be high. This tracing would suggest that the patient is awake during the initial hours of the recording. This point is further supported by frequent changes in body position as seen in the top row occurring at the same time. In this case, use of actigraphy would result in a lower estimate of total sleep time and, therefore, higher AHI.

be seen in any patient, but may be more problematic in patients with a severe tremor. Such patients may, therefore, be suboptimal candidates for portable monitoring. In **Fig. 10**, the episode of movement is followed by what is scored by the monitor's internal algorithm as a hypopnea. However, there is no associated oxyhemoglobin desaturation and certainly no EEG data to support

that this event is indeed a hypopnea. The event may also simply represent mouth breathing. Therefore, interpretation of machine-scored events should be done with caution by experienced and specialty-trained personnel. Although most type 3 monitors cannot confirm arousals or awakenings because of the lack of EEG data, peripheral arterial tonometry, which measures vasoconstriction

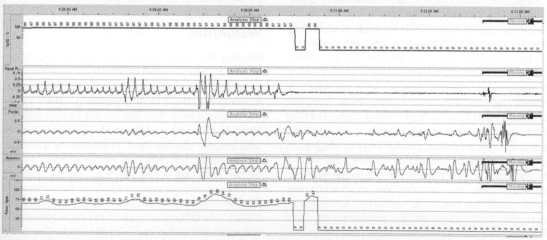

Fig. 9. Loss of data. The nasal airflow channel shows complete cessation in flow, which could be mistaken for an apneic event. Both the oxyhemoglobin saturation and heart rate show values of zero, indicating the loss of data.

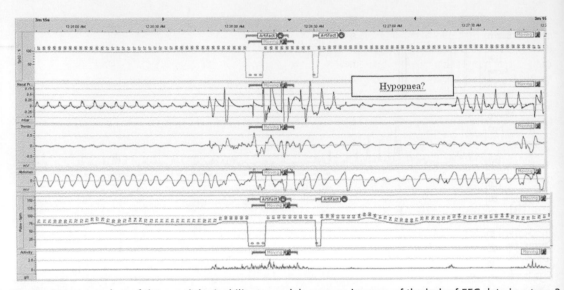

Fig. 10. Movement, loss of data, and the inability to mark hypopnea because of the lack of EEG data in a type 3 recording. This figure shows irregular breathing effort based on abdominal and chest movement. Activity on actigraphy is also increased, followed by transient loss of data with the heart rate and oxyhemoglobin desaturation dropping to zero. Thus, loss of data may be secondary to movement of the oximeter, which measures both oxyhemoglobin saturation and heart rate. This episode of movement is followed by what appears to be a hypopnea. However, there is no associated oxyhemoglobin desaturation or available EEG data indicating the presence of an arousal to score this event as a hypopnea. The event may also simply represent mouth breathing.

through a finger sensor, has been shown to have good correlation with subcortical arousals and apneas seen in standard polysomnography.[18] This technology may allow scoring of RERAs, but it has not been specifically validated for this purpose.[19]

Other limitations to portable monitors exist. The lack of an available technician hampers the ability to ensure high-quality signal acquisition during the recording. If severe OSA is present, prompt, same-night CPAP titration could not be performed, as would occur in an in-laboratory study. Rather, the patient will require a second study. However, some split-CPAP titration studies may comprise insufficient time to adequately determine an optimal CPAP pressure, and an additional titration study may not be avoidable. Although most patients may have a better night of sleep at home, patients with psychophsyiologic insomnia are more likely to have restful sleep outside of their home environment; studies performed on these patients may, therefore, produce higher diagnostic yield if they are performed in the sleep laboratory. Home studies may miss important incidental findings that may be detected on an in-laboratory PSG, such as nocturnal seizures, arrhythmias, periodic limb movements, parasomnias, and RERAs.[20]

Little data on the cost-effectiveness of portable monitors is available, and more studies are clearly

needed. An Australian study comparing the use of home portable monitors to in-laboratory polysomnography for the diagnosis of OSA and CPAP titration in a high-risk population found the portable-monitoring arm to be significantly more cost-effective at 3 months.[21] However, the portable-monitoring arm involved practitioner visits, whereas the latter arm involved physician visits. Although unattended studies are generally more convenient for patients, they may also necessitate an additional trip to the hospital if in-person orientation is required.

VALIDATION

Studies that have examined concurrent polysomnography and portable testing have found a significant correlation between AHIs of both testing modalities in the laboratory setting, rather than in the home, where they are meant to be used.[22,23] The sleep heart health study compared home unattended studies with in-laboratory polysomnography and found that home studies yielded higher respiratory disturbance indices (RDIs) in patients with less severe OSA as determined by PSG and lower RDIs in patients with more severe OSA.[24] No difference was found between median values of both studies.[24] A pilot study conducted by Kuna[6] showed a decreased correlation between portable testing and polysomnography when the former is conducted in the home as compared to portable and full sleep studies conducted in the laboratory. Comparisons between these two modalities do not take into account night-to-night variability. Multiple night recordings are needed to take into account night-to-night variability when comparing home portable testing to in-laboratory polysomnography.[6] Studies that have compared in-laboratory polysomnography with home portable diagnostic testing plus CPAP auto-titration have found no difference in outcomes measures, such as CPAP adherence and quality of life.[21,22,25–27] Many of these studies examined a highly selective group of patients with a high pretest probability of sleep apnea who lacked comorbidities.

FUTURE DIRECTIONS

Portable sleep studies may be very useful because of their convenience, relative ease of application, and the lack of requirement of a technologist in attendance. However, these monitors carry specific indications and limitations. More controlled studies are needed to determine whether overall clinical outcomes and economics of portable management pathways are at least equivalent to traditional pathways, which have required the use of in-laboratory services for diagnosis and treatment initiation. As technological advances in this arena continue to be made at a remarkable pace, the design and development of these new monitors must be supported by thoughtfully designed research that guides the sleep practitioner in the effective application of these devices.

REFERENCES

1. Young T, Palta M, Dempsey J, et al. The occurrence of sleep-disordered breathing among middle-aged adults. N Engl J Med 1993;328:1230–5.
2. Services. Centers for Medicare & Medicaid. Decision memo for continuous positive airway pressure (CPAP) therapy for obstructive sleep apnea; CAG-00093R2. Available at: https://www.cms.hhs.gov/mcd/viewdecisionmemo.asp?id=227. Accessed March 3, 2009.
3. Services. Centers for Medicare & Medicaid. Decision memo for sleep testing for obstructive sleep apnea; CAG-00405N. Available at: https://www.cms.hhs.gov/mcd/viewdecisionmemo.asp?id=227. Accessed March 3, 2009.
4. Ferber R, Millman R, Coppola M, et al. Portable recording in the assessment of obstructive sleep apnea. ASDA standards of practice. Sleep 1994; 17:378–92.

5. Chesson AL Jr, Berry RB, Pack A. Practice parameters for the use of portable monitoring devices in the investigation of suspected obstructive sleep apnea in adults. Sleep 2003;26:907–13.
6. Kuna ST. Portable-monitor testing: an alternative strategy for managing patients with obstructive sleep apnea. Respir Care 2010;55:1196–215.
7. Collop NA, Anderson WM, Boehlecke B, et al. Clinical guidelines for the use of unattended portable monitors in the diagnosis of obstructive sleep apnea in adult patients. Portable Monitoring Task Force of the American Academy of Sleep Medicine. J Clin Sleep Med 2007;3:737–47.
8. Bar A, Pillar G, Dvir I, et al. Evaluation of a portable device based on peripheral arterial tone for unattended home sleep studies. Chest 2003;123:695–703.
9. Elbaz M, Roue GM, Lofaso F, et al. Utility of actigraphy in the diagnosis of obstructive sleep apnea. Sleep 2002;25(5):527–31.
10. Mayer P, Pepin JL, Bettega G, et al. Relationship between body mass index, age and upper airway measurements in snorers and sleep apnoea patients. Eur Respir J 1996;9:1801–9.
11. Lam B, Ip MS, Tench E, et al. Craniofacial profile in Asian and white subjects with obstructive sleep apnoea. Thorax 2005;60:504–10.
12. Calleja JM, Esnaola S, Rubio R, et al. Comparison of a cardiorespiratory device versus polysomnography for diagnosis of sleep apnoea. Eur Respir J 2002;20:1505–10.
13. Iber C, Ancoli-Israel S, Chesson AL, et al; for the American Academy of Sleep Medicine. AASM manual for the scoring of sleep and associated events: rules, terminology, and technical specifications. 1st edition. Westchester (IL): American Academy of Sleep Medicine; 2007. p. 45–7.
14. Oksenberg A, Silverberg DS, Arons E, et al. Positional vs nonpositional obstructive sleep apnea patients: anthropomorphic, nocturnal polysomnographic, and multiple sleep latency test data. Chest 1997;112:629–39.
15. Quintana-Gallego E, Villa-Gil M, Carmona-Bernal C, et al. Home respiratory polygraphy for diagnosis of sleep-disordered breathing in heart failure. Eur Respir J 2004;24:443–8.
16. Randerath W. Treatment options in Cheyne-Stokes respiration. Ther Adv Respir Dis 2010;4(6):341–51.
17. Flemons WW, Littner MR, Rowley JA, et al. Home diagnosis of sleep apnea: a systematic review of the literature. An evidence review cosponsored by the American Academy of Sleep Medicine, the American College of Chest Physicians, and the American Thoracic Society. Chest 2003;124:1543–79.
18. Penzel T, Fricke R, Jerrentrup A, et al. Peripheral arterial tonometry for the diagnosis of obstructive

sleep apnea. Biomed Tech (Berl) 2002;47(Suppl 1 Pt 1):315–7.

19. O'Donnell CP, Allan L, Atkinson P, et al. The effect of upper airway obstruction and arousal on peripheral arterial tonometry in obstructive sleep apnea. Am J Respir Crit Care Med 2002;166:965–71.

20. Gay PC, Selecky PA. Are sleep studies appropriately done in the home? Respir Care 2010;55:66–75.

21. Antic NA, Buchan C, Esterman A, et al. A randomized controlled trial of nurse-led care for symptomatic moderate-severe obstructive sleep apnea. Am J Respir Crit Care Med 2009;179:501–8.

22. Michaelson PG, Allan P, Chaney J, et al. Validations of a portable home sleep study with twelve-lead polysomnography: comparisons and insights into a variable gold standard. Ann Otol Rhinol Laryngol 2006;115:802–9.

23. Su S, Baroody FM, Kohrman M, et al. A comparison of polysomnography and a portable home sleep study in the diagnosis of obstructive sleep apnea syndrome. Otolaryngol Head Neck Surg 2004;131:844–50.

24. Iber C, Redline S, Kaplan Gilpin AM, et al. Polysomnography performed in the unattended home versus the attended laboratory setting–Sleep Heart Health Study methodology. Sleep 2004;27:536–40.

25. Berry RB, Hill G, Thompson L, et al. Portable monitoring and autotitration versus polysomnography for the diagnosis and treatment of sleep apnea. Sleep 2008;31:1423–31.

26. Whitelaw WA, Brant RF, Flemons WW. Clinical usefulness of home oximetry compared with polysomnography for assessment of sleep apnea. Am J Respir Crit Care Med 2005;171:188–93.

27. Mulgrew AT, Fox N, Ayas NT, et al. Diagnosis and initial management of obstructive sleep apnea without polysomnography: a randomized validation study. Ann Intern Med 2007;146:157–66.

Current Published Standards Including Centers for Medicare and Medicaid Services Requirements for Portable Monitoring

Nancy Collop, MD

KEYWORDS

- CMS • Polysomnography • Out of center sleep testing
- Portable monitoring • NCD • LCD

Obstructive sleep apnea (OSA) is a common disorder in which the upper airway repetitively narrows and/or collapses during sleep, resulting in hypoxemia and sleep disruption. The confirmation of the disorder to date has required a diagnostic study during sleep that monitors the necessary physiologic signals. Before 2009, most insurance companies and the Centers for Medicare and Medicaid Services (CMS) mandated that polysomnography in a sleep laboratory be performed to diagnose OSA in both adults and children. Polysomnography typically includes monitoring of sleep stage by electroencephalography, electro-oculography, and chin electromyography; cardiac signals via electrocardiography; respiratory effort and flow; oxygen saturation; and leg movements via leg electromyography. Polysomnography provides extensive information about the patient's sleep and sleep-disordered breathing, and other sleep disorders can be determined during the test.

Interest in developing less intensive diagnostic testing for OSA has been ongoing for many years. Because the diagnosis of OSA is based on symptoms and breathing indices during sleep, many investigators and companies have worked on developing devices that are simple and could be used in the home. The advantages of such devices include home-based, testing which is more convenient for the patient, and potentially lower cost (if successful).

In 1994, the American Sleep Disorders Association (ASDA) published its first paper on this subject in which it examined 23 published papers on portable monitoring devices.[1] In that review, the first categorization scheme for diagnostic sleep testing was unveiled and classified devices into 4 levels. Level 1 was standard in-laboratory, attended polysomnography; level 2, comprehensive, unattended polysomnography done outside the sleep laboratory; level 3, modified portable sleep apnea testing that measures at least 4 channels; and level 4, continuous single-bioparameter or dual-bioparameter recording. Although these distinctions were made, use of these devices for diagnostic testing (levels 2, 3, 4) was not recommended at that time. Although that original article used the term level, many subsequent articles have used the term type to describe this schema. A practice parameter issued by the ASDA in 1997 entitled *Practice Parameters for the Indications for Polysomnography and Related Procedures* reviewed level 3 and 4 devices but, again, did not suggest broad usage for these devices.[2] In 2003, the American Academy of Sleep Medicine (AASM; formerly the ASDA), the American College of Chest Physicians, and the American Thoracic Society collaborated to publish a series of papers that examined the evidence supporting the use of portable diagnostic devices.[3–6] The comprehensive evidence review used the method published

Emory University, 1841 Clifton Road, WWHC Room 502, Atlanta, GA 30329, USA
E-mail address: nancy.collop@emory.edu

Sleep Med Clin 6 (2011) 367–374
doi:10.1016/j.jsmc.2011.05.003
1556-407X/11/$ – see front matter © 2011 Published by Elsevier Inc.

sleep.theclinics.com

by Sackett and colleagues[7] to assign evidence levels to the chosen literature. In that review, they examined 51 articles (1990–2001) and again divided the analysis into the ASDA types (1–4). The accompanying practice parameter outlined the recommended usage for portable monitoring devices, which again was limited. CMS was asked to specifically review the use of portable testing devices for the diagnosis of OSA in 2004 to 2005. They did not adopt a change in their requirements for laboratory-based polysomnography (type 1) based on the trisociety evidence review and their own internal review.[8]

In 2007, CMS was again asked by the American Academy of Otolaryngology to review the use of portable devices for OSA. In rulings released in 2008 to 2009,[9] they ultimately allowed the use of portable monitoring devices. In 2007, the AASM also published clinical guidelines for the use of portable monitoring devices and many of the stipulations in that document were used by CMS in their ruling.[10] In 2010, Canada released its own standards for use of portable monitors and, in 2011, the AASM released new accreditation standards for sleep centers and other diagnostic testing entities for out-of-center sleep testing in adults. This article reviews the important elements of the current published standards for diagnostic testing using portable monitors.

AASM CLINICAL GUIDELINES FOR PORTABLE MONITORING

The current guideline published in 2007 provides information about the indications, technology and methodology.[10] It was based on review of papers from 1997 to 2006 (37 papers). It also used data gathered in the evidence reviews about sensors from the AASM Scoring Manual and associated papers.[11]

Indications

The guidelines point out that the patient populations that had been evaluated with portable monitors were typically highly selected (ie, had a high pretest probability for OSA). Most of the studies excluded patients with significant comorbidities, and the populations were usually middle-aged, and predominantly male. Therefore, the recommendations were based on excluding patients who fell outside those parameters. In addition, most studies were conducted by physicians and researchers knowledgeable about OSA. **Box 1** summarizes the indications for use of portable monitoring as outlined by the AASM clinical guidelines paper. In summary, the patients who are considered to be appropriate for use of PM must

---

Box 1
AASM clinical guidelines for portable monitoring

1. When diagnosing OSA, portable monitoring devices should only be used in conjunction with a comprehensive sleep evaluation by a board-certified or board-eligible sleep medicine specialist.
2. Provided that #1 has been performed, PM may be used as an alternative to in-laboratory PSG for diagnosing OSA but only in patients with a high pretest probability of having moderate to severe OSA.
3. PM is not appropriate in patients with significant comorbid medical conditions (severe pulmonary, cardiac, or neuromuscular disease) because the presence of those conditions may result in inferior accuracy of PM.
4. Use of PM is not appropriate for patients suspected of having other sleep disorders (central sleep apnea, periodic limb movement disorder, insomnia, parasomnias, circadian rhythm disorders, or narcolepsy).
5. PM should not be used for general screening of asymptomatic populations.
6. PM may be indicated for the diagnosis of OSA in patients who might not be able to obtain in-laboratory PSG because of immobility, safety, or critical illness.
7. PM may be indicated to monitor responses to alternative treatments for OSA (oral appliances, surgery, weight loss).

Adapted from Collop NA, Anderson WM, Boehlecke B, et al. Clinical guidelines for the use of unattended portable monitors in the diagnosis of obstructive sleep apnea in adult patients. J Clin Sleep Med 2007;3(7):737–47; with permission.

---

be at high risk for OSA based on an assessment of pretest probability, and not have comorbid medical disorders or comorbid sleep disorders. Because PM have only been tested for patients with OSA, other types of sleep disorders still require in-laboratory polysomnography. In addition, because the patients are considered to have a high probability for OSA, a negative test should prompt an in-laboratory polysomnogram (PSG).

Technology

The taskforce found that the prior level/type classification did not provide enough granularity to be useful in evaluation of the technology. Instead, they attempted to review devices based on type of signal: (1) oximetry; (2) respiratory monitoring; (3) cardiac monitoring; (4) measures of sleep/wake activity; and (5) body position. The recommended sensors for PM mirrored those used in polysomnography (**Table 1**).

Table 1
AASM clinical guidelines for portable monitoring: recommended sensors

Sensor	Measurement	Comments
Nasal pressure transducer	Airflow	Needed for hypopneas, flow limitation
Oronasal thermistor	Airflow	Needed for apneas
Respiratory inductance plethysmography	Effort	Maybe be calibrated or uncalibrated
Pulse oximeter	Oxygen saturation	Needs adequate sampling rate, signal averaging time, and accommodation for motion artifact

Adapted from Collop NA, Anderson WM, Boehlecke B, et al. Clinical guidelines for the use of unattended portable monitors in the diagnosis of obstructive sleep apnea in adult patients. J Clin Sleep Med 2007;3(7):737–47; with permission.

Methodology

A summary of the recommended methodology is given in **Box 2**. Because PM studies are usually done by sleep specialists, the AASM taskforce considered that some specific expertise should be present to assure adequate knowledge on the methods of performing PM. Because AASM accreditation requires high and consistent standards, the guideline recommended that PM should be performed under the auspices of an AASM-accredited comprehensive sleep medicine program. In addition, the literature supported a higher level of accuracy if manual scoring or manual editing of automated scoring by skilled personnel was used, therefore this was also recommended, with subsequent review of the raw data by a sleep specialist (preferably board certified or eligible in sleep medicine). Recommendations regarding specific scoring criteria note that it should be consistent with published criteria.

Summary of AASM Clinical Guideline

The recommendations in this guideline include that a patient being considered for a portable monitoring test be evaluated by a health care provider knowledgeable about OSA who can determine that the patient has a high probability for having significant (moderate to severe) OSA, does not have significant comorbid disorders that would reduce the accuracy of the device, and do not have coexistent sleep disorders. The study should be done with a device that measures flow, effort, and oximetry; can display raw data that can be manually scored or edited; and interpreted by a specialist who is sleep medicine board certified/eligible. The patient should be followed after the study to review results, which, if negative, should lead to in-laboratory polysomnography.

CMS GUIDELINES

There are 3 types of policies that CMS provides: National Coverage Provisions, National Coverage Determinations (NCD), and Local Coverage Determinations (LCD). NCDs apply to all CMS

Box 2
AASM clinical guidelines for portable monitoring: recommended methodology

1. PM testing should be done within AASM-accredited sleep centers. There should be policies and procedures for application, scoring, and interpretation of PM as well as quality/performance improvement program.
2. An experienced sleep technician/technologist or appropriately trained health care practitioner must apply the PM sensors or educate the patient about the correct application.
3. PM devices must have display of raw data for manual scoring or the ability to edit automated scoring; this should be performed by a trained and qualified sleep technician/technologist. A board-certified/eligible sleep specialist should review the raw data.
4. Scoring criteria should be performed using the current AASM standards.
5. Because of false-negative PM tests, in-laboratory polysomnography should be performed In cases in which PM is technically inadequate or does not make a diagnosis of OSA.
6. A follow-up visit with a physician or physician extender should be performed on all patients undergoing PM to discuss the results of the test.

Adapted from Collop NA, Anderson WM, Boehloecke B, et al. Clinical guidelines for the use of unattended portable monitors in the diagnosis of obstructive sleep apnea in adult patients. J Clin Sleep Med 2007;3(7):737–47; with permission.

Table 2
Sample LCDs on HST

LCD	State	Posted	Policy
National Government Services (L26428)	CT	1/1/11	1. Diagnosis of OSA can be made using in-laboratory PSG or type II, III, or IV[a] devices 2. Acceptable codes: 95800, 95801, 95806, G0398, G0399, and G0400 (must measure respiratory movement, airflow, and oxygen saturation) 3. Not covered for patients with certain comorbidities including moderate to severe pulmonary disease, neuromuscular disease affecting muscles of respiration, congestive heart failure, and suspicion of the presence of other sleep disorders
Highmark (L27530)	DE	1/3/11	1. OSA can be diagnosed using full in-laboratory PSG or unattended home sleep monitoring using type II, type III, or type IV[a] devices 2. Screening tests, in the absence of associated signs, symptoms, or complaints will be denied 3. Devices must be FDA approved 4. HST can be used to diagnose OSA if "the HST is reasonable and necessary for the diagnosis of the patient's condition, meets all Medicare requirements, and the physician who performs the service has sufficient training and experience to reliably perform the service" 5. HST should be performed over a period of 3 consecutive nights to acquire quality data; however, multiple nights of HST are considered as 1 study 6. Acceptable codes: 95800, 95801, 95806, G0398, G0399 and G0400 7. OSA (327.23) is the only acceptable diagnosis for HST
Palmetto GBA L28292	CA	1/7/11	1. HST devices must be FDA approved type II, type III, or type IV with at least 2 channels using actual recorded hours of sleep 2. HST must be interpreted by (1) ABSM-certified physician; (2) ABMS sleep-certified physician; (3) physician who has completed an ABMS-approved residency or fellowship training and meets sleep medicine examination requirements; or (4) physician with active membership of sleep center or laboratory accredited by AASM or JC 3. Acceptable codes: 95800, 95801, 95806, G0398, G0399, G0400 4. Acceptable ICD-9 diagnosis codes are the same for HST as for in-laboratory PSG and MSLT
Wisconsin Physicians Service Insurance Corporation (L31082)	IA	12/17/10	1. HST devices measuring ≥3 channels that include actigraphy, oximetry, and peripheral arterial tone are covered when used to aid the diagnosis of OSA in beneficiaries who have signs and symptoms that indicate OSA if performed unattended in or out of a sleep laboratory facility or attended in a sleep laboratory facility 2. Codes 95800, 95801 and 95806 are allowed when performed in a facility. Codes G0398, G0399 and G0400 are allowed when performed in the home 3. HST is covered only for diagnosis of OSA 4. HST must be interpreted by (1) ABSM-certified physician; (2) ABMS sleep-certified physician; or (3) physician with active membership of sleep center or laboratory accredited by AASM or JC 5. Technician must be an RPSGT (through BRPT) or a CPFT, RPFT, CRT, or RRT (through NBRC) 6. Allowed ICD-9 codes: 327.23 (OSA), 780.53 (hypersomnia with sleep apnea) and 780.54 (hypersomnia) 7. HST must be performed using Medicare-approved devices 8. More than 1 HST per year is not expected

(continued on next page)

Table 2
(continued)

LCD	State	Posted	Policy
Noridian Administrative Services, LLC (L24350)	AZ	11/21/10	1. Unless performed according to the CMS NCD, HST will be denied in the home setting except when performed with a technician in attendance and when it conforms to all other data and sleep staging criteria for coverage 2. HST must be interpreted by (1) ABSM-certified physician; (2) ABMS sleep-certified physician; (3) physician who has completed an ABMS-approved residency or fellowship training and meets sleep medicine examination requirements; or (4) physician with active membership of sleep center or laboratory accredited by AASM or JC 3. Acceptable codes: 95806, G0398, G0399, G0400 4. Acceptable ICD-9 diagnosis codes are the same for HST as for in-laboratory PSG and MSLT
First Coast Service Options, Inc. (L29949)	FL	11/21/10	1. To perform the technical component of HST, the center or laboratory must maintain documentation of accreditation through AASM or JC 2. HST must be interpreted by: (1) ABSM-certified physician; (2) ABMS sleep-certified physician; (3) ABFM-certified physician with certificate of added qualifications in sleep medicine; or (4) physician with active membership of sleep center or laboratory accredited by AASM or JC 3. HST can be followed by in-laboratory PSG if the result of an HST is insufficient (case-by-case basis). Persuasive evidence justifying the medical necessity of additional testing is required 4. Acceptable codes: G0398, G0399, G0400 5. Acceptable ICD-9 diagnosis codes are the same for HST as for in-laboratory PSG and MSLT, with some exceptions 6. Appropriate certification for technicians and technologists is required 7. HST can be billed (technical and professional components) by a board-certified sleep physician not affiliated with an accredited center if the physician is office based
Trailblazer Health Enterprises, LLC (L28640)	CO	1/1/11	1. Physician performing service must be (1) ABSM-certified physician; (2) ABMS sleep-certified physician; or (3) physician with active membership of sleep center or laboratory accredited by AASM or JC 2. HST must be done "in conjunction with a comprehensive sleep evaluation and in patients with a high pretest probability of moderate to severe obstructive sleep apnea" 3. HST is not covered "for persons with comorbidities…other symptoms…or for screening asymptomatic persons" 4. HST must be interpreted by "a physician or doctoral level professional with satisfactory training in sleep medicine and significant experience in interpretation of standard polysomnograms" 5. Acceptable codes: G0398, G0399, G0400 6. Allowed ICD-9 codes are 327.23 (OSA), 780.51 (insomnia with sleep apnea), 780.53 (hypersomnia with sleep apnea), and 780.57 (unspecified sleep apnea)

Abbreviations: ABMS, American Board of Medical Specialties; ABSM, American Board of Sleep Medicine; BRPT, Board of Registered Polysomnographic Technologists; CPFT, Certified Pulmonary Function Technician; CRT, Certified Respiratory Therapist; FDA, US Food and Drug Administration; ICD, International Classification of Diseases; JC, Joint Commission; MSLT, Mean Sleep Latency Test; NBRC, National Board for Respiratory Care; RPFT, Registered Pulmonary Function Technician; RPSGT, Registered Polysomnographic Technician; RRT, Registered Respiratory Therapist.

[a] Type IV devices must measure 3 channels.

jurisdictions and can be found at the following Web site: http://www.cms.gov/center/coverage.asp. NCDs provide information on broad coverage or noncoverage. LCDs are the contractor-developed coverage policies and are usually developed to cover appropriate use of new technology; address services with an abuse history or the potential for abuse; or high-volume, high-cost services. The most recent NCD for diagnostic testing for OSA was released on 3/3/09 (240.4.1). This NCD was the first to allow the use of home sleep tests to diagnose sleep apnea. It was developed after the Agency for Health Research and Quality (AHRQ) sponsored 2 reviews, a Technology Assessment and another entitled *OSAHS: Modeling Diagnostic Strategies*. The difference between these assessments and prior assessments done by CMS is that these analyses included studies in which outcomes with home sleep testing (HST) devices were compared with polysomnography with the primary consideration being CPAP adherence. At the time, there were 2 studies that concluded that it did not matter which way a person was tested.[12,13] Once CMS decided to proceed with HST, they next needed to determine which types of devices were acceptable and what was the appropriate patient population. Because there were no CPT codes available for some of the HST devices, they also needed to develop codes. The only CPT codes for HST at the time were 95806 and 95807. Code 95806 had the following definition: "sleep study, simultaneous recording of ventilation, respiratory effort, electrocardiogram or heart rate, and oxygen saturation, unattended by a technologist," with 95807 differing by the modifier that it was "attended." This was for a type III device only. On further evaluation, this code was changed to the following: "sleep study, simultaneous recording of heart rate, oxygen saturation, respiratory airflow, and respiratory effort (eg, thoracoabdominal movement) unattended by a technologist." In addition, both G and T (temporary) codes were added. The T codes were made into permanent codes in January 2011.

NCD 240.4.1 used the same type 1 to 4 descriptions as used in the original ASDA document, with the exception of type 4 devices. In the NCD, type 4 devices could have 1, 2, or 3 parameters.

NCD 240.4.1 Nationally Covered Indications

For testing for OSA only, type 1 (in-laboratory polysomnography), type 2, and type 3 devices, both attended and unattended, are covered. Type 4 devices are covered only if they measure 3 channels, one of which is airflow; or devices that measure actigraphy, oximetry, and peripheral arterial tone.

LCD Information

There are multiple LCDs that also address testing for OSA. Many have the same elements as each other, but some are different. The major differences relate to who can perform or interpret the tests and which codes should be used. Some also address accreditation status for sleep laboratories. A summary of some of the current LCDs can be seen in **Table 2**.

CPAP

Because CPAP is the most common and effective treatment of OSA, its prescription is intricately intertwined with the diagnostic testing. The NCD for use of CPAP (240.4) further differentiates how HST can be used to qualify a patient for a CPAP device. The most recent version was clarified on October 15, 2008. Consistent with the diagnostic testing, it allows for in-laboratory PSG, unattended PSG, and home sleep tests meeting the criteria as outlined earlier. It goes on to state that, in order for patients to qualify for CPAP, they must meet the following criterion using the Apnea-Hypopnea Index (AHI) or Respiratory Disturbance Index (RDI):

1. AHI or RDI greater than or equal to 15 events per hour of sleep or continuous monitoring, respectively, or
2. AHI or RDI greater than or equal to 5 and less than or equal to 14 events per hour of sleep or continuous monitoring, respectively, with documented symptoms of excessive daytime sleepiness, impaired cognition, mood disorders or insomnia, or documented hypertension, ischemic heart disease, or history of stroke.

The AHI is equal to the average number of episodes of apnea and hypopnea per hour of sleep. The RDI is equal to the average number of respiratory disturbances per hour of continuous monitoring.

It goes on to clarify that, "if the AHI or RDI is calculated based on less than 2 hours of continuous recorded sleep, the total number of recorded events to calculate the AHI or RDI during sleep testing is at least the number of events that would have been required in a 2-hour period."

AASM OUT-OF-CENTER ACCREDITATION STANDARDS

In January 2011, the AASM adopted new standards for entities wishing to use out-of-center diagnostic testing for OSA. These standards closely parallel the clinical guidelines,[10] but not completely. Like the other standards that the AASM uses for sleep centers, these standards

Table 3
AASM mandatory standards for OCST accreditation in adults

#	Standard	Brief Description
A-1	Facility license	Must maintain valid license to provide health care services
A-2	Medical code of ethics	Must follow the AMA Code of Medical Ethics
B-1	MD	Must have a physician serving as a single medical director with valid state license
B-2	MD qualifications	A physician who is Sleep Medicine board certified (ABMS, ABSM, AOA) or board eligible
B-3	MD responsibilities	Responsible for oversight of testing; qualifications of personnel, and quality assurance program
B-4	MD CME	Participate in 10 CME credits/y in sleep medicine
B-5	IP	Must have valid license in all states in which interpretations are performed
B-6	IP qualifications	A physician who is Sleep Medicine Board certified (ABMS, ABSM, AOA) or board eligible
B-7	IP CME	Participate in 10 CME credits/y in sleep medicine
B-12	OCST on-call coverage	Must provide nighttime on-call coverage by medical director or licensed sleep board physician or appropriately trained personnel
G-1	Patient management	Must perform a follow-up visit on all patients undergoing OCST to discuss results and treatment options. If not provided by the entity, must have an existing relationship with an AASM-accredited sleep center
G-4	PAP titration during OCST	PAP titration or other therapy initiated by the OCST entity must be done in accordance with AASM practice parameters
G-6	PAP assessment	Patients prescribed PAP by OCST entity must offer follow-up PAP assessment within 12 weeks of therapy initiation

Abbreviations: AMA, American Medical Association; AOA, American Osteopathic Association; CME, continuing medical education; IP, interpreting physician; MD, medical director; OCST, out-of-center sleep testing; PAP, positive airway pressure.
Available from: http://www.aasmnet.org/resources/pdf/OCSTstandards.pdf.

include sections on personnel, including the medical director, interpreting physicians, technical personnel, and scoring personnel; patient acceptance criteria; facility and equipment; policy and procedures; protocols; equipment maintenance; data acquisition, scoring, and reports; patient evaluation and management; records; and quality assurance/improvement. Fourteen of the standards are considered mandatory, and those are listed in **Table 3**. The medical director and interpreting physicians are all required to be physicians who are board certified or board eligible in sleep medicine and maintain continuing medical education credits. The technical personnel who instruct patients do not have to have a degree unless required by state law; however, the scoring personnel should have some additional training in sleep medicine.

The equipment used must meet one of the current HST codes, and protocols have to be in place for cleaning and inspecting the equipment.

There are recommendations about what the reports must contain and that the physician must have the ability to review raw data.

The accreditation requires a follow-up visit to review the test results, and a management plan. If the out of center sleep testing (OCST) itself is not doing the management, then they must have a documented relationship with an AASM-accredited center. The OCST must have a quality assurance program that, at a minimum, tracks test failure and retest rates.

SUMMARY

Diagnostic testing for OSA is moving into a new era in which many patients will be tested in their homes rather than in the sleep centers. Physicians performing such testing should be versed in the practice of sleep medicine so that they can appropriately choose which patients can be accurately diagnosed with such testing; understand the types of devices, including their individual pros and cons; how to perform, score, and interpret these tests; and recommend treatment options. They must develop algorithms for such testing that include what to do with negative tests (true or false negatives), inadequate tests, or unexpected results. There will be challenges with bringing such testing to mainstream medicine in the United States, but the process has already begun.

REFERENCES

1. Ferber RA, Millman RP, Coppola MP, et al. ASDA standards of practice: portable recording in the assessment of obstructive sleep apnea. Sleep 1994;17:378–92.

2. American Sleep Disorders Association. Practice parameters for the indications for polysomnography and related procedures: Polysomnography Task Force, American Sleep Disorders Association Standards of Practice Committee. Sleep 1997;20:406–22.

3. Flemons W, Littner M, Rowley J, et al. Home diagnosis of sleep apnea: a systematic review of the literature. An evidence review cosponsored by the American Academy of Sleep Medicine, the American College of Chest Physicians, and the American Thoracic Society. Chest 2003;124:1543–79.

4. Chesson AL Jr, Berry RB, Pack A. Practice parameters for the use of portable monitoring devices in the investigation of suspected obstructive sleep apnea in adults. Sleep 2003;26:907–13.

5. ATS/ACCP/AASM Taskforce Steering Committee. Executive summary on the systematic review and practice parameters for portable monitoring in the investigation of suspected sleep apnea in adults. Am J Respir Crit Care Med 2004;169:1160–3.

6. Flemons W, Littner M. Measuring agreement between diagnostic devices. Chest 2003;124:1535–42.

7. Sackett DL, Strauss SE, Richardson WS, et al. Evidence based medicine: how to practice and teach EBM. 2nd edition. Edinburgh (UK): Churchill Livingstone; 2000.

8. Lux L, Boehlecke B, Lohr K; RTI International. Effectiveness of portable monitoring devices for diagnosing obstructive sleep apnea: Update of a Systematic Review. Available at: https://www.cms.gov/coverage/download/id110e.pdf. Accessed July 1, 2011.

9. Available at: http://www.cms.gov/center/coverage.asp. Accessed July 1, 2011.

10. Collop N, Anderson M, Boehloecke B, et al. Clinical guidelines for the use of portable monitoring in adult patients. J Clin Sleep Med 2007;3(7):737–47.

11. Iber C, Ancoli-Israel S, Chesson AL Jr, et al, American Academy of Sleep Medicine. The AASM manual for the scoring of sleep and associated events: rules, terminology and technical specifications. 1st edition. Oakbrook (IL): AASM; 2007.

12. Whitelaw WA, Brant RF, Flemons WW. Clinical usefulness of home oximetry compared with polysomnography for assessment of sleep apnea. Am J Respir Crit Care Med 2005;171:188–93.

13. Mulgrew A, Fox N, Ayas N, et al. Diagnosis and initial management of obstructive sleep apnea without polysomnography. Ann Intern Med 2007;146:157–66.

Portable Recording in the Diagnosis and Management of Sleep-Disordered Breathing: Unanswered Questions and Future Research

Philip R. Westbrook, MD[a,b,c,d,e,*]

KEYWORDS

- Portable • Diagnosis • Sleep • Breathing • Apnea

"The unifying principle is really quite simple; it is that we are in this business to serve people and that means not only maintaining and restoring their health, but doing it without violating the budget they are willing to pay."
—David M. Eddy[1]

"The best interest of the patient is the only interest to be considered—."
—William J. Mayo in 1910 commencement address, Rush Medical College, Chicago, IL.

Sleep-disordered breathing, particularly obstructive sleep apnea/hypopnea, is a prevalent human affliction.[2,3] It is as common as asthma or diabetes, and like those conditions is a chronic disease. The potential for sleep-related upper airway collapse is a birthright of our species, a price we pay for the evolution of speech[4]; however, it probably was not a significant problem until the invention of farming some 13,000 years ago. Rather suddenly there was surplus food, calories that allowed

a favored few to become obese. In the last century, the increasing availability of relatively inexpensive high-calorie food has led to an epidemic of obesity in many countries.[5] Now almost everyone in North America can overeat, with the resultant challenge to the patency of the sleeping pharyngeal passageway. It is estimated that one-third of the population of the United States is obese, that about 10% have obstructive sleep apnea (OSA), and that 25% of those have moderate to severe disease as measured by the frequency of abnormal breathing events (Apnea/Hypopnea Index or AHI). Of these, an estimated 93% of women and 83% of men remain undiagnosed.[6]

The examination of the sleeping patient has, from the rediscovery of sleep apnea in 1965, been primarily a laboratory-based test. This initially made a lot of sense. We observed with fascination that some individuals stopped breathing as soon as they fell asleep. Some fell asleep and could not breathe in spite of strenuous attempts to do so. A few fell asleep and would not try to breathe.

Disclosure: See last page of article.
a Department of Medicine, Mayo Clinic College of Medicine, Rochester, MN, USA
b Department of Medicine, David Geffen School of Medicine, UCLA, Los Angeles, CA, USA
c Advanced Brain Monitoring, Inc, 2237 Faraday Avenue, Suite 100, Carlsbad, CA 92008, USA
d Watermark Medical, Inc, 1750 Clint Moore Road, Suite 101, Boca Raton, FL 33487, USA
e Ventus Medical, Inc, 1301 Shoreway Road, Suite 425, Belmont, CA 94002, USA
* Advanced Brain Monitoring, Inc, 2237 Faraday Avenue, Suite 100, Carlsbad, CA 92008.
E-mail address: philip@westbrooks.com

Sleep Med Clin 6 (2011) 375–385
doi:10.1016/j.jsmc.2011.05.008

Once we started looking at what happened under the cover of darkness, we found other abnormalities, from periodic movement of limbs to violent movements of the whole body. Sleep was not just one, but two previously unexplored states of existence. Learning what could happen in those states required the recording of sleep electrophysiologically. We obviously had much to learn about what happened during this time of supposed "rest."

Until about 20 years ago, machines to record the electroencephalogram (EEG), the electrooculogram (EOG), the electromyogram (EMG), and all the other physiology we wanted to examine were huge. They were ink-spewing monsters that ate trees and required trained technicians to keep them running. These technicians also became expert at applying to the patient the many sensors we thought were necessary to give us the information we thought we needed. Polysomnography was born, and with it, polysomnographic technicians and polysomnographers (now called sleep medicine specialists), clustered mostly in academic sleep centers. A new medical specialty was created, with its own organization, and with all the benefits and consequences that medical guilds engender.

Medical specialties such as sleep medicine develop from a knowledge base gained by research and experience, but in the United States, medical reimbursement is largely generated by procedures. The singular procedure in sleep medicine that has funded the rapid growth of the field is the attended in-laboratory polysomnography (PSG). The payment for this complex and costly procedure has been generous enough, and the demand for sleep apnea diagnostic testing high enough, to lead to a rapid increase in the number of investor-owned sleep laboratories. It has also made sleep medicine an economically attractive area for practice and contributed greatly to the growth of the specialty practice.

Over the past 10 years, advances in technology have allowed the miniaturization of recorders and have led to portable wearable devices that can be used for focused data acquisition in any location. The need for readily available, less-expensive, and more patient-friendly alternatives to PSG for diagnosing sleep-disordered breathing (SDB) has prompted the development of numerous systems for portable recording or "monitoring" (PM) in the patient's home. The development of auto-adjusting continuous positive airway pressure (CPAP) machines that negate the routine necessity of in-laboratory manual titration of CPAP pressure,[7] and the very recent decision by the Centers for Medicare and Medicaid Services to reimburse for PM,[8,9] has made PM a potentially viable alternative to PSG. This has threatened a revolution in sleep

medicine and, as in all revolutions, there are opposing sides. The organization representing sleep specialists, now the American Academy of Sleep Medicine (AASM), has been less than enthusiastic about the possibility that portable focused recording for SDB would become the standard practice, and the corollary that the diagnosis and management of uncomplicated patients with SDB would become the province of the primary care physician team.[10] Patient advocacy groups, on the other hand, have supported the use of new approaches to the diagnosis of sleep apnea and its management.[11]

Although I am not aware of any published data, my estimate from talking to colleagues running clinical sleep laboratories is that more than 90% of PSGs are done for the confirmation of suspected SDB or for CPAP titration in patients diagnosed as having OSA. The clinical sleep specialist's concern is that laboratory-attended PSG, the procedure upon which the specialty has been based, could become like the use of maggots for wound debridement—ancient technology, occasionally useful, but seldom required.

There are a number of excellent recent reviews of focused recording for SDB and its use in a pathway of disease management.[12–18] I did not attempt to duplicate them here.

In this article, I explore some of the questions surrounding portable recording and what future research might be required to answer these questions. In so doing I question the evidence that the PSG remains necessary for the routine clinical diagnosis of SDB. By diagnosis I mean the determination of just 3 things: (1) Is sleep-disordered breathing present? (2) If so, what kind is it? (3) How bad is it?

I did not reference the old division of portable monitors (actually portable recorders, because no person is in attendance to view the signals as they are being recorded) into 4 levels developed by the American Sleep Disorders Association (ASDA, precursor of the AASM) Standards of Practice Committee in the early 1990s.[19] This is because technology, and recent reimbursement guidelines, has made them obsolete. Instead, I posit a hypothetical portable device, the hypothetical focused recorder (HFR), that meets the spirit if not quite all the letters of the AASM recommendations for portable recording technology.[15] The term "hypothetical focused recorder" is used to indicate one type of portable recording device, whereas the terms "portable monitor" (PM) and "home sleep test" (HST) are used interchangeably.

I use the term "value" in addressing research needs, and by value I mean health outcomes per dollar spent. Achieving high value in health care is what is "in the best interest of the patient." Indeed, as Porter points out, "This goal is what matters for patients and unites the interests of all actors in the system. If value improves, patients, payers, providers, and suppliers can all benefit while the economic sustainability of the health care system increases."[20(p1)]

THE HYPOTHETICAL FOCUSED RECORDER

The HFR is a hypothetical portable diagnostic device that records airflow by nasal pressure, oxyhemoglobin saturation, and pulse rate with a pulse oximeter with the appropriate signal averaging time, respiratory effort, position, movement (actigraphy), and snoring. It has firmware that continuously monitors recording quality and can notify the patient if the placement of the nasal cannula or the oximeter needs adjustment. It can be easily and reliably self-applied by the patient with simple instructions. The study failure rate in clinical use is less than 5%. The device can record at least 2 nights with a single battery charge. It provides a full disclosure recording of all signals. The recording is automatically scored for behavioral sleep and abnormal breathing events, but is fully editable by a sleep technologist and a sleep physician. The scoring algorithms are fully explained. The procedure for downloading and uploading data is simple and quick, as is preparation of the device for its next use.

Actually there are now available a number of portable recording systems that meet or exceed all or most of the specifications of the HFR. I am not saying that all the things the HFR records are necessary for the diagnosis of SDB, only that they match the information about breathing recorded by the typical laboratory PSG.[21] The HFR also includes all the attributes rated as necessary or desirable in portable recording systems for SDB by an unscientific survey of sleep medicine experts.[22] What they do not do of course, is to record sleep electrophysiologically.

The presently accepted purpose of measuring the AHI in OSA is to provide one numerical measure of the severity of the physiologic disorder of breathing. No matter how the AHI is obtained there is conflicting evidence as to what level of physiologic abnormality results in proven sequelae. Although it is now accepted that severe obstructive apnea merits treatment because of its proven health consequences, the definition of "true positive" disease is still debatable. Much research remains to be done because limited outcomes data exist on the value of detecting and treating patients with a mild or borderline AHI.

The questions outlined in the following section, many unanswered or incompletely answered, include those previously raised by a number of thoughtful reviewers of this subject.[16–18,23,24] Some of the questions are philosophic or political, and defy purely scientific answers. My list is in no particular order, is quite personal, and is certainly not exhaustive.

QUESTIONS AND RESEARCH NEEDS
Is Recording the EEG, EOG, and Submental EMG, the Sleep Montage, Really Necessary for Diagnosing SDB?

There are basically 3 reasons usually given to support the necessity for recording of the typical sleep montage when recording for the diagnosis of sleep apnea. They are that it is required for use as the denominator when calculating the AHI, that it is needed to measure arousals, and that it is necessary to identify rapid-eye movement (REM) sleep.

Is it necessary to measure sleep electrophysiologically to get a meaningful AHI?
The standard metric for severity of SDB remains the AHI, although it is variably defined and poorly related to outcomes such as abnormal sleepiness.[25–28] The AHI is calculated as the total number of apneas plus hypopneas experienced by a patient during a study divided by that patient's sleep time. Because patients almost never spend the entire recording time asleep, the AHI calculated using unadjusted total recording time as the denominator will be less than the AHI calculated using sleep time.

There are a number of things that make it very unlikely that we will think someone is asleep when he or she is really awake. The HFR can take advantage of the fact that our species does not sleep randomly throughout the 24-hour day, but tends to have a consolidated major sleep period at night. So the patient is instructed to wear the HFR in bed at night. Humans sleep lying down, and during sleep we are relatively quiescent—we don't move around much. However, we are not quiet, especially if we are one of those we would consider testing for sleep apnea. Snoring is a reliable indicator of sleep. During sleep, people exhibit varying degrees of inspiratory flow limitation, whereas during wakefulness the resting inspiratory flow curve appears sinusoidal. Of course during apneas and hypopneas the person being recorded is asleep.

There are also clues to someone being awake, including it being daytime, an upright position, sustained movement, the sinusoidal inspiratory flow tracing, absence of snoring, and variable respiratory and heart rates.

Actigraphy (wrist) has been examined in 3 studies and has been shown to estimate actual sleep time with reasonable accuracy.[29–31] Combining actigraphy with other signs of sleep, such as snoring and flow limitation, could further improve estimation of sleep time. Douglas and colleagues[32] looked at the need for usual PSG recording in 200 consecutive adults referred for PSG, most for suspected OSA, and determined that the AHI calculated using recording time was just as useful as that calculated using EEG sleep time. They concluded that recording sleep electrophysiologically was without diagnostic value and that sleep apnea could be as accurately defined by AHI using time in bed as the denominator as by AHI calculated using time asleep.

By editing the HFR full-disclosure recording in a very commonsense way, the total recording time can be reduced to an estimated sleep time that should be close to the real sleep time. Furthermore, the overestimation of the denominator in calculating AHI may not make much difference for clinical purposes. In a recording of 7 hours where the sleep time is overestimated by an hour and the "true" AHI is 83, the AHI calculated by recording time would be 71, hardly a clinically important difference. At the other end of event frequency where the total number of events is 25, calculating the AHI using 7 and 6 hours time both give an AHI of 4.

Further research on the value of including electrophysiologically determined sleep time in the routine diagnostic portion of a management pathway for patients suspected of having SDB might be helpful. However, in the recent study by Berry and colleagues,[33] there was no statistically significant difference in AHIs calculated using electrophysiologic and behavioral sleep times.

Is it necessary to measure sleep electrophysiologically to identify EEG arousals, or will other arousal indicators suffice?

Two AASM criteria for scoring hypopneas require the ability to score an arousal.[21] Arousals can be defined by respiratory, behavioral, and autonomic changes as well as by EEG markers. Indeed, such EEG arousal surrogates may be more reliably measured and be more closely associated with daytime consequences.[34–36] For example, respiratory effort–related arousals or flow limitation events are quite easily recognized by a plateau in inspiratory flow contour, a small dip in saturation, terminated suddenly by a change in snoring, a resumption of sinusoidal flow, an increase in pulse rate, and often a movement.[36,37] Oximetry can be analyzed for pulse wave amplitude changes that are evidence of autonomic arousal.[38]

Further research is needed on which arousal metrics, if any, provide the best value for prediction of daytime health consequences. This would seem to be true not only in the management of a patient's SDB, but also for evaluating the impact of other sleep-disturbing conditions.

Is it necessary to measure sleep electrophysiologically to identify REM sleep?

The simple answer is that yes, it is necessary if it is important to be absolutely sure that during a period of recording the patient is in REM sleep. However, it is not established how important clinically distinguishing REM from non-REM sleep is. The clinical importance of REM-predominant OSA is still controversial.[39,40] Identifying periods of REM sleep on the full-disclosure HFR is usually possible by noting the timing and pattern of the fall in oxyhemoglobin saturation and/or the onset of obstructive events unaccounted for by a change in position. There is currently no sleep stage–specific treatment for OSA, so staging sleep seems unlikely to affect patient outcomes.

Patients with OSA occurring only in REM sleep are rather rare, and the value of identifying REM-only sleep apnea needs further research.

What Needs to Be Recorded to Confidently Diagnose Sleep-Disordered Breathing?

The HFR records lots of things. Are they all necessary to confirm the diagnosis of SDB? Most of the randomized clinical trials showing equivalent outcomes to PSG used limited channel recorders based just on oximetry alone, or oximetry and either snoring or autonomic arousals.[33,41–44] Only one so far has used a diagnostic recording device like the HFR.[45] However, those randomized in these studies came from a cohort of patients at high risk for OSA and most had rather extensive exclusion criteria to eliminate potentially confounding conditions. It would make sense that patients at quite high risk for significant oxygen desaturation with obstructive events, for example patients who are obese, old, have preexisting lung disease, or who live in Denver or Calgary, could be adequately confirmed with overnight oximetry alone. However, patients at marginal risk, such as young skinny females studied at or near sea level, eg, Stanford, might need the more complete set of measurements offered by the HFR to identify subtle flow-limitation events.

It may be that the one-size-fits-all approach we have used in the past is no longer appropriate, and that portable recording for confirming SDB in selected patients could become even more highly focused and simple. Research on the value of this approach is needed.

What Needs to Be Recorded to Confirm Efficacy of Non-CPAP Treatment of SDB?

This question is obviously related to the one just prior. Once sleep apnea that warrants treatment has been diagnosed, what needs to be recorded to objectively confirm that the treatment is working?[46] CPAP units can now record not only time-on-pressure but also flow limitation event frequency and mask leaks. This objective evidence of success is not built into other treatment options. Weight loss, position restriction, mandibular advancing appliances, the expiratory positive pressure device (Provent; Ventus Medical Inc., Boca Raton, FL, USA), and the various surgical procedures are all therapies that should be objectively evaluated for outcome in each patient in whom they are tried. The AASM has endorsed portable recording for this purpose. However, it is not known if the same information thought to be needed for diagnosis of SDB is also required for the evaluation of treatment success. For example, it might be that just a recording of snoring, position, and oximetry with sufficient accuracy, along with symptomatic improvement, would confirm the success or failure of treatment of OSA with an oral device or with Provent.

Lowering the respiratory disturbance index (RDI) is only one of the measures of treatment efficacy. Success in management of this lifetime disease will require long-term data acquisition and collation of meaningful patient health outcomes.[47] Agreement on outcome measures for the management of patients with OSA is required before the value of any management pathway can be assessed. This will require further research.

What Is Normal or Abnormal Breathing During Normal Sleep Conditions?

What is an abnormal average amount of SDB for a person sleeping where and when they usually sleep? Stated another way, what is pathologic SDB and how is it best defined? Comparing 2 different approaches to the diagnosis of OSA is problematic if there are no agreed on diagnostic criteria. The metric historically used is a measure of event frequency during sleep, usually in the laboratory on a single night; however, the type of event to be counted, and how often those events need to occur to trigger intervention, remains controversial. Probably the most common threshold of abnormal is an apnea/hypopnea associated with a 4% desaturation index of 5 or more. This threshold of abnormality is applied to adults regardless of age, sex, or ethnicity, and absent much evidence that it is clinically relevant. The fact that some epidemiologic studies show that an AHI of 5 or 10 is associated with a trivial rise in blood pressure, does not mean that a 60-year-old Hispanic female without otherwise explained daytime sleepiness or other risk factors needs a CPAP prescription if her AHI is 5. Is an average AHI of 16 in a healthy asymptomatic 70-year-old white male abnormal? A recent study of super-healthy subjects found an average RDI in those older than 65 was 22.0 (SD ± 17.4).[48]

Research is needed to determine what defines the disease or diseases we call sleep apnea and if there is asymptomatic but clinically important (worth finding because it is bad for the person and it can be successfully treated) OSA.

Should Only Those Patients with a High Pretest Probability for Moderate to Severe OSA Have a Portable Focused Recording for SDB Confirmation?

The latest AASM task force on portable recording recommends that only patients at high pretest probability for moderate to severe OSA (as determined by a sleep specialist) are candidates for portable studies.[15] Most would agree that patients at no or very low risk for SDB do not need a test, be it PSG or HST, for a disease that they are very likely not to have. In the same vein it could be argued that a patient at very high risk be just started on treatment.[23,49] It is the patients in the low-risk and middle-risk categories that are the problem. The truth is that, short of examining how well they breathe at night, we have no reliable way of identifying them. Most patients with sleep apnea, if defined by an AHI of 5 or more, have an AHI in the mild range, between 5 and 20.

Future research on the value of PM should include subjects with a high pretest probability of mild OSA.

What Comorbidities Should Exclude Patients from Having a Diagnostic Study with a Portable Recorder?

The AASM answer to this question is as follows: *PM is not appropriate for the diagnosis of OSA in patients with significant comorbid medical conditions that may degrade the accuracy of PM, including, but not limited to, moderate to severe pulmonary disease, neuromuscular disease, or congestive heart failure.*[15(p740)] This recommendation was based on the lack of portable recorder outcome studies that included patients with the named conditions. But there is no logical reason to exclude patients with pulmonary disease from having a diagnostic study with an HFR unless they are on prescribed nocturnal supplemental oxygen or need to be sleep attended. To my knowledge, a nasal cannula for recording pressure has not been proven to work with a nasal cannula that is being used to deliver oxygen, so these patients should have attended monitoring if one is going to substitute a pressure-measuring cannula for an oxygen-delivering cannula. If a patient with neuromuscular disease is able to apply the portable monitor and normally sleeps unattended at home, there is no reason why the study cannot be done with the HFR unattended at home. The same reasoning applies to patients with heart disease, including congestive heart failure. The knowledgeable physician (or techni-cian) can identify the pattern of Cheyne-Stokes breathing on an HFR recording as well as on a PSG record. Patients with preexisting chronic stable pulmonary disease and ventilation/perfu-sion abnormalities are the ones most likely to have their OSA accurately diagnosed by nocturnal oximetry alone.[50] Any condition that "may degrade the accuracy of PM" will also degrade the accu-racy of pattern recognition on a PSG recording.

If patients are sleeping unattended at home and are physically and mentally capable of reliably self-applying the recorder, and no same-night inter-vention is planned, why exclude them? There is no risk from the recorder or its sensors.

Future research on the value of PM should include all patients at risk for all levels of OSA severity regardless of comorbidities.

Is a PM Focused on the Diagnosis of SDB Inadequate for Diagnosing Other Sleep Disorders?

A criticism of PM for SDB frequently voiced is that it is not helpful in the evaluation of other sleep disorders, and that the full panoply of sensors offered by PSG allows the physician to find these unsuspected and presumably treatable problems. The AASM guide-lines are as follows: *PM is not appropriate for the diagnostic evaluation of OSA in patients suspected of having other sleep disorders, including central sleep apnea, periodic limb movement disorder (PLMD), insomnia, parasomnias, circadian rhythm disorders, or narcolepsy.*[15(p740)] This is a bit like saying that the problem with a tennis court is that it is not a suitable place to play football. That is true, but irrelevant. The game being played, as stated in the introductory paragraphs, is "Diagnose Sleep-Disordered Breathing." The claim that central sleep apnea cannot be diagnosed with an HFR is simply untrue. Central sleep apnea events are as easily

detected on the HFR recording as on a PSG recording. Both require breathing pattern recognition.

Insomnia and circadian rhythm disorders are not indications for either PM or a PSG. Narcolepsy needs an overnight documentation of sleep before a Multiple Sleep Latency Test, but the overnight recording by itself is not a diagnostic test for this disorder. A suspected REM Sleep Behavior Disorder or seizure disorder currently certainly does require attended videotaped full PSG with potential extra EEG monitoring, but these are uncommon diagnostic dilemmas unlikely to be confused with typical SDB.

One of the most frequently stated arguments against portable recording is that it will not detect periodic limb movements in sleep (PLMS). It is true that the HFR will usually not pick up PLMS, but this fact could be used as an argument in favor of portable recording. Evidence for the diagnostic or functional significance of asymptomatic PLMS is lacking, and finding it could lead to unnecessary treatment.[51,52] Occult periodic limb movements, which are movements unknown to the patient (except perhaps by bed-partner report), not asso-ciated with Restless Legs Syndrome, and detected only electrophysiologically, are very common.[53] In the study of super-healthy asymptomatic individ-uals older than 65, the average Periodic Limb Movement Index was 20.2 per hour with 1 standard deviation being 32.3![48] Periodic leg movements, like excess nose hair and wrinkles, appear to be a normal accompaniment of aging.

Further research on the value of detection of asymptomatic PLMS in patients suspected of having SDB is needed.

Should Portable Monitoring Be Used for Screening for SDB in an Asymptomatic Population?

The AASM Task Force on Portable Monitoring states that "PM is not appropriate for general screening of asymptomatic populations."[15(p740)] However, given the prevalence of sleep apnea, and that it appears to be a risk factor for cardiovas-cular and metabolic disease, and that perhaps 30% of those with moderate to severe sleep apnea are not sleepy, an argument could be made that at least certain subsets of the asymptomatic population should have their breathing during sleep examined. The population might be the same as those now recommended to have a test for colon cancer, or perhaps males whose age and body mass index are both over 35. What we do not know is if early detection of SDB in asymptomatic males could lead to cost-effective treatment and prevention of downstream health consequences. Until we do, use of PM for screening for OSA probably should not be recommended.

Research on the value of screening certain high-risk but asymptomatic populations should be supported.

What Is the Real Cost of an Attended In-Laboratory PSG Versus the Real Cost of a Focused Home Recording?

Cost is a critical issue, one about which there are precious few hard data. It is difficult to imagine that a home self-applied HFR would be as expensive to perform as an attended in-laboratory PSG, but no actual real-life cost comparisons have yet been published with an HFR-type portable system used in patients at all risk levels. There have been 3 theoretical models published. Chervin and colleagues[54] modeled the cost-utility of 3 approaches to the diagnosis of sleep apnea and treatment (CPAP): laboratory attended PSG for diagnosis and CPAP titration, HST for diagnosis but attended laboratory CPAP titration, and empirical therapy with CPAP. The outcome was quality-adjusted life years for the first 5 years after diagnosis ($QUALY_5$). Chervin and colleagues[54] concluded that, in spite of the increased costs, under the modeled conditions the laboratory PSG for diagnosis is the preferable and most cost-effective path when compared with the other 2 options. A similar analysis comparing the cost-effectiveness of full-night PSG for diagnosis and CPAP prescription, split-night PSGs, and HST with CPAP automated titration was published in 2006.[55] Both of these modeling studies assumed high baseline prevalence of patients with moderate to severe OSA, and low specificity for the HST. The calculated gain in QUALY for the full PSG approach versus HST in the study by Deutsch and colleagues[55] was small and cost $6500. A recent economic decision model by Ayas and colleagues[56] presented formulae by which they determined the pretest probability above which it would be appropriate to use portable studies to rule in OSA in symptomatic patients. With their model and its assumptions, the pretest probability of a symptomatic patient having OSA would need to be greater than 0.68 for HST to be a better buy economically than a split-night PSG. The mathematical models presented in these 3 studies are interesting but totally dependent on the assumptions used, and all presume that the pattern of respiratory changes recorded in the home are less reliable than those measured in the laboratory. Furthermore, none of the models took into account the number of

patients at high risk for OSA referred for PSG who never show up for their test because of inconvenience or cost.

In all real-life studies where costs of home versus laboratory diagnosis have been estimated, the pathway to treatment using PM has been significantly less expensive. White and colleagues[57] found that the analysis time for a rather complex PM system was significantly less, by more than 1 hour on average, than PSG, but no actual cost comparison was made. Fletcher and colleagues,[58] in a study of 63 patients, estimated the costs of using a home test for OSA and auto adjusting CPAP for determination of therapeutic pressure, and found it was less than one-quarter of the cost of a laboratory approach. In a study of 55 patients at high risk for OSA who received focused home sleep studies either set up by a technician in the patient's home or self-applied by the patient, there was agreement, determined by the decision of whether or not to treat with CPAP, between the PM and PSG in 76% of cases.[59] The total estimated costs of the PM set up by the technician was about 65% of the PSG cost, but the self-applied PM cost was 90% of the PSG cost because of HST failures, mostly unreadable airflow signals.

The most intriguing published study to date that includes a measurement of costs is that of Antic and colleagues.[43] They used overnight oximetry results as well as symptoms to identify patients referred to academic sleep disorders centers with suspected OSA as being at high risk for moderate to severe disease. The exclusion criteria were reasonable with only about 6% of those assessed for eligibility being rejected on medical grounds. Patients (n = 195) were randomized to 1 of 2 care models. Patients in the Model A arm going to automated positive airway pressure (APAP) titration at home, CPAP commencement at fixed pressure, and care supervised under a protocol by nurse specialists experienced in the care of patients on CPAP. Patients randomized to Model B had their entire care directed in the traditional way by sleep medicine physicians, including a diagnostic PSG, in-laboratory CPAP titration, commencement of a fixed CPAP, and follow-up as decided by the physician. Within-study resource use and costs were carefully recorded. The nurse-led model of care demonstrated 3-month outcomes that were not inferior to the physician-directed care in every way examined (Epworth Sleepiness Scale, Maintenance of Wakefulness Test, objective CPAP adherence, Functional Outcomes of Sleep Questionnaire, Short-Form 36 Health Survey, executive neuro-cognitive function, and patient satisfaction) while being significantly less costly by $A1,111 per patient.

There are now 6 randomized clinical trials (RCTs) comparing home versus laboratory management pathways with a total of 945 patients at risk for moderate to severe OSA.[33,41–46] None of the studies showed any outcome advantage of the traditional laboratory PSG pathway over one based on home studies and APAP. Two of the trials included a comparison of the costs of the alternate management routes, but so far the results of only one have been published.[43]

The Veterans Sleep Apnea Treatment Trial (VSATT), a large 2-site RCT evaluating the functional outcome and costs of home management of patients with OSA, has thus far been analyzed only for outcomes and published only as an abstract.[45] However, this clinical trial demonstrated noninferiority of outcomes following 3 months of CPAP treatment in patients with OSA randomized to either standard in-laboratory PSG testing or home testing with an HFR-type portable system.

The obvious implication is that focused home testing and home CPAP initiation is effective in treating OSA. As has been noted by others, costs must include all those incurred on the path to treatment. The real cost of a test must be known before its value can be calculated. If PM is less expensive, then the burden of proof that the laboratory PSG is a preferred pathway for management of the typical patient rests with its advocates. However, determining cost is probably the easier part of the value equation. I think determining what we should measure for outcome, and then how we should measure it, is much more difficult.

The cost of the PM/APAP management pathway for patients with OSA needs further research so its value can be ascertained.

Should Primary Care Physicians Be Allowed to Use PM?

The medical society representing sleep specialists and responsible for accrediting sleep disorder centers has been rather adamant that only sleep specialists working in accredited sleep-disorder centers are qualified to order and perform PM.[15] This consensus opinion is unsupported by evidence that allowing the non–sleep specialist physician to perform an HFR will have adverse consequences. Many generalists now successfully manage chronic diseases, such as hypertension, asthma, and diabetes, with the occasional help from a specialist for patients with particularly complex problems. A recent study demonstrated that a simplified less-costly nurse-led model of

care had the same results as physician specialist–directed care in the management of symptomatic moderate to severe OSA.[43]

One of the concerns expressed by sleep specialists is that letting a patient's primary care-giver diagnose and treat sleep apnea will lead to overuse of PM. However, this is really a concern about the medical reimbursement system in the United States, not a concern about the value of the test itself. Also, the concern about overuse can be equally applied to specialists and PSG. There are few if any impediments to self-referral of patients for PSG on the part of those who own or are employed by sleep laboratories. Although it is possible for payers to require "screening" tests, such as Sleep Apnea Clinical Score or others that predict risk of disease and severity, and to require preapproval for those below a certain risk threshold, the tests can be manipulated by unscrupulous patients or providers.

Because standard recommended practice is to refer all patients suspected of having SDB to a sleep specialist, the primary care physician has little reason to learn about the diagnosis and treatment of OSA. The AASM recommendations based on the inadequate training of the primary care physician thus become a self-fulfilling prophecy.

What is needed is a concerted effort by all stakeholders, including equipment manufacturers and vendors, as well as sleep specialists, the AASM, and the American Association of Sleep Technologists, to provide the primary care physician with the resources and knowledge to manage the typical patient with clinically important OSA over that patient's lifetime. The resources include trained team members, physician extenders experienced in sleep medicine, who will provide most of the care. I think this will not be an easy sell. The economic and emotional investment in sleep laboratories is huge, and the threat to that investment is real. Yet there is no reason why sleep specialists cannot evolve to embrace PM as the value path to OSA diagnosis and focus on the really difficult problem: treatment.

Research is needed to measure the value of having a patient's primary care provider be able to order a confirmatory test for his or her patient with suspected sleep apnea.

Should Portable Recorders Be Standardized?

The fact that there are a number of different portable recorders available with considerable variations in hardware and measurement methods is a criticism leveled at them. However, the same criticism could be made of PSG systems, which remain equally unstandardized in terms of respiratory recording. The AASM has made recommendations about PM technology,[15] opting to apply the AASM recommendations for in-laboratory sensors to PM in spite of the fact that an unattended home recording has its own set of requirements, including reliability and ease of use. Standardization of systems has definite advantages in research applications but can stifle innovation. I would vote no. The better PM will always be invented next year, and what would be most helpful is a requirement that their proponents provide validation studies establishing their appropriate use and value in the intended patient population.

Can a Portable Recording Be Used to Rule Out (Exclude) as Well as Rule in (Include) Disease?

The AASM recommendation assumes that portable recording cannot rule out SDB.[15] However, recent studies have shown that portable recording can both confirm and exclude the diagnosis of SDB.[55,56] Clearly, a portable device that provides a full-disclosure recording of the same breathing parameters as a laboratory PSG can record normal breathing as well as abnormal breathing. In fact, a 2-night recording in the home might be a better way of establishing the absence of significant SDB than a single-night laboratory PSG, assuming we could define clinically important SDB. Current AASM recommendations are that if a person at risk for OSA has a "negative" but technically valid portable recording, that person should have a laboratory PSG. Allowing for night-to-night variability in SDB, it is not clear what the PSG is going reveal about that patient's breathing that the HFR study did not. If that same patient has a negative but technically valid PSG, should the patient have a portable recorder study? Probably the patient should start with a sleep medicine consult.

One major problem is that we are still unsure of what defines the disease. The use of a single AHI threshold with or without a complaint of sleepiness does not make sense. As noted previously, we really do not know what the normal spread of apnea/hypopnea event frequency is, and sleepiness is both an ubiquitous and nonspecific symptom. It is possible that sleep apnea is a disease that can be defined only by response to treatment. Unfortunately, treatment is difficult, and some important responses, eg, longer survival or more QUALYs, may take years to become apparent.

Perhaps we need a long-term large population epidemiologic study of the value of detecting and treating as best possible mild-to-moderate SDB, including asymptomatic OSA.

SUMMARY

Diagnosing the usual patient suspected of having sleep apnea is easy. For those who cannot be diagnosed in the waiting room, recent evidence suggests portable focused recording works as well as PSG and is less expensive. Questions remain, and further research is needed to define the value of focused home recording in the diagnosis and management of patients with possible SDB.

DISCLOSURE

The author is an employee and board member of and shareholder in Advanced Brain Monitoring, Inc, a sleep-related medical device research and development company. He is an employee (retainer) of and consultant to and shareholder in Watermark Medical, Inc, a company that markets home diagnostic testing for sleep-disordered breathing. He is a consultant to Ventus Medical, Inc, a company that has developed and markets a treatment for obstructive sleep apnea. He is an employee (retainer) of and consultant to Rotech, Inc, a durable medical equipment company that also provides home diagnostic testing for sleep-disordered breathing. He is one of the inventors of the ARES portable sleep apnea diagnostic system developed by Advanced Brain Monitoring, Inc, and used by Watermark Medical and Rotech.

REFERENCES

1. Eddy DM. Preface. In: Eddy DM, editor. Clinical decision making: from theory to practice: a collection of essays from The Journal of the American Medical Association. London: Jones and Bartlett Publishers; 1996. p. xi–xii.
2. Young T, Palta M, Dempsey J, et al. The occurrence of sleep-disordered breathing among middle-aged adults. N Engl J Med 1993;328(17):1230–5.
3. Duran J, Esnaola S, Rubio R, et al. Obstructive sleep apnea-hypopnea and related clinical features in a population-based sample of subjects aged 30 to 70 yr. Am J Respir Crit Care Med 2001;163(3pt1): 685–9.
4. Fogal RB, Malhotra A, White DP. Sleep 2: pathophysiology of obstructive sleep apnoea/hypopnea syndrome. Thorax 2004;59:159–63.
5. Ogden C, Carroll MD, Curtin LR, et al. Prevalence of overweight and obesity in the United States, 1999–2004. JAMA 2006;295(13):1549–55.
6. Young T, Evans L, Inn L, et al. Estimation of the clinically diagnosed proportion of sleep apnea syndrome in middle-aged men and women. Sleep 1997;20(9):705–6.

7. Cross MD, Vennelle M, Engleman HM, et al. Comparison of CPAP titration at home or the sleep laboratory in the sleep apnea hypopnea syndrome. Sleep 2006;29(11):1451–5.

8. Decision Memo for Continuous Positive Airway Pressure (CPAP) Therapy for Obstructive Sleep Apnea (OSA). (CAG-00093R2). Centers for Medicare & Medicaid Services; 2008.

9. Decision Memo for Sleep Testing for Obstructive Sleep Apnea (OSA). (CAG-00405N). Centers for Medicare and Medicaid Services; 2008.

10. Epstein LJ, Silber MH. AASM response to the ASAA letter to the editor [letter to the editor]. J Clin Sleep Med 2006;2(3):363–4.

11. Grandi E. An open letter to the sleep community and physicians concerned with sleep-disordered breathing [letter to the editor]. J Clin Sleep Med 2006;2(3):361–2.

12. Flemons WW, Littner MR, Rowley JA, et al. Home diagnosis of sleep apnea: a systematic review of the literature. An evidence review cosponsored by the American Academy of Sleep Medicine, the American College of Chest Physicians and the American Thoracic Society. Chest 2003;124(4):1543–79.

13. Trikalinos TA, Ip S, Raman G. Agency for Healthcare Research and Quality. Technology Assessment: Home diagnosis of obstructive sleep apnea-hypopnea syndrome. 2007. Available at: http://www.cms.hhs.gov/deterinationprocess/dowloads/id48TA.pdf. Accessed May 14, 2011.

14. Ahmed M, Patel P, Rosen I. Portable monitors in the diagnosis of obstructive sleep apnea. Chest 2007; 132:1672–7.

15. Collop NA, Anderson WM, Boehlecke B, et al. Portable Monitoring Task Force of the American Academy of Sleep Medicine: clinical guidelines for the use of portable monitors in the diagnosis of obstructive sleep apnea in adult patients. J Clin Sleep Med 2007;3(7):737–47.

16. Collop NA. Portable monitoring for the diagnosis of obstructive sleep apnea. Curr Opin Pulm Med 2008;14:525–9.

17. Kuna ST. Portable-monitor testing: an alternative strategy for managing patients with obstructive sleep apnea. Respir Care 2010;55(9):1196–215.

18. Sunwoo B, Kuna T. Ambulatory management of patients with sleep apnea: is there a place for portable monitor testing? Clin Chest Med 2010; 31(2):299–308.

19. Ferber R, Millman R, Coppola M, et al. ASDA Standards of Practice: portable recording in the assessment of obstructive sleep apnea. Sleep 1994;17(4): 378–92.

20. Porter Perspective ME. What is value in health care? N Engl J Med 2010;363:2477–81.

21. Iber C, Ancoli-Israel S, Chesson AL, et al. The AASM manual for the scoring of sleep and associated events. American Academy of Sleep Medicine; 2007.

22. Westbrook PR. Survey regarding limited diagnostic systems for sleep apnea. J Clin Sleep Med 2007; 3(3):318–20.

23. Phillips B. Improving access to diagnosis and treatment of sleep-disordered breathing. Chest 2007; 132:1418–20.

24. Ross SD, Sheinhait IA, Harrison KJ, et al. Systematic review and meta-analysis of the literature regarding the diagnosis of sleep apnea. Sleep 2000;23(4):1–14.

25. Redline S, Budhiraja R, Kapur V, et al. The scoring of respiratory events in sleep: reliability and validity. J Clin Sleep Med 2007;3(2):169–200.

26. Kapur VK, Baldwin CM, Resnick HE, et al. Sleepiness in patients with moderate to severe sleep-disordered breathing. Sleep 2005;28(4):472–7.

27. Flemons WW, Buysse D, Redline S, et al. Sleep-related breathing disorders in adults: recommendations for syndrome definition and measurement techniques in clinical research. The Report of an American Academy of Sleep Medicine Task Force. Sleep 1999;22:667–89.

28. Ruehland WR, Rochford PD, O'Donoghue FJ, et al. The new AASM criteria for scoring hypopneas: impact on the apnea hypopnea index. Sleep 2008; 32(2):150–7.

29. Hedner J, Pillar G, Pittman SD, et al. A novel adaptive wrist actigraphy algorithm for sleep-wake assessment in sleep apnea patients. Sleep 2004; 27(8):1560–6.

30. Elbaz M, Roue GM, Lofaso F, et al. Utility of actigraphy in the diagnosis of obstructive sleep apnea. Sleep 2002;25(5):525–9.

31. Wang D, Wong KK, Dungan GC II, et al. The validity of wrist actimetry assessment of sleep with and without sleep apnea. J Clin Sleep Med 2008;4(5): 450–5.

32. Douglas N, Thomas S, Jan MA. Clinical value of polysomnography. Lancet 1992;339(8789):347–50.

33. Berry RB, Hill G, Thompson L, et al. Portable monitoring and autotitration versus polysomnography for the diagnosis and treatment of sleep apnea. Sleep 2008;31(10):1423–31.

34. Catcheside PG, Orr S, Chiong SC, et al. Noninvasive cardiovascular markers of acoustically induces arousal from non-rapid-eye-movement sleep. Sleep 2002;25(7):67–74.

35. Stepanski EJ. The effect of sleep fragmentation on daytime function. Sleep 2002;25(3):268–78.

36. Johnson PL, Edwards N, Burgess KR, et al. Detection of increased upper airway resistance during overnight polysomnography. Sleep 2005;28(1):85–90.

37. Ayappa I, Norman MS, Krieger AC, et al. Non-invasive detection of respiratory effort-related arousals (RERAs) by nasal cannula/pressure transducer system. Sleep 2000;23:763–71.

38. Pitson DJ, Stradling JR. Autonomic markers of arousal during sleep in patients undergoing investigation for obstructive sleep apnoea, their relationship to EEG arousals, respiratory events and subjective sleepiness. J Sleep Res 1998;7:53–9.

39. Haba-Rubio J, Janssens JP, Rochat T, et al. Rapid eye movement related disordered breathing: clinical and polysomnographic features. Chest 2005;128: 3350–7.

40. Chervin RD, Aldrich MS. The relation between multiple sleep latency test findings and the frequency of apneic events in REM and non-REM sleep. Chest 1998;113:980–4.

41. Whitelaw WA, Brant RF, Flemons WW. Clinical usefulness of home oximetry compared with polysomnography for assessment of sleep apnea. Am J Respir Crit Care Med 2005;171:188–93.

42. Mulgrew AT, Fox N, Ayas NT, et al. Diagnosis and initial management of obstructive sleep apnea without polysomnography: a randomized validation study. Ann Intern Med 2007;146:157–66.

43. Antic NA, Buchan C, Esterman A, et al. A randomized controlled trial of nurse-led care for symptomatic moderate–severe obstructive sleep apnea. Am J Respir Crit Care Med 2009;179:501–8.

44. Skomro RP, Gjevre J, Reid J, et al. Outcomes of home-based diagnosis and treatment of obstructive sleep apnea. Chest 2010;138(2):257–63.

45. Kuna ST, Maislin G, Hin S, et al. Non-inferiority of functional outcome in ambulatory management of obstructive sleep apnea. Am J Respir Crit Care Med 2010;181:A5560.

46. Pack AI, Gurubhagavatula I. Economic implications of the diagnosis of obstructive sleep apnea. Ann Intern Med 1999;130(6):533–4.

47. Lee TH. Perspective: putting the value framework to work. N Engl J Med 2010;363:2481–3.

48. Pavlova MK, Duffy JF, Shea SA. Polysomnographic respiratory abnormalities in asymptomatic individuals. Sleep 2008;31(2):241–8.

49. Senn O, Brack T, Russi EW, et al. A continuous positive pressure airway trial as a novel approach to the diagnosis of the obstructive sleep apnea syndrome. Chest 2006;129:67–75.

50. Douglas NJ. Sleep-related breathing disorder. 3. How to reach a diagnosis in patients who may have the sleep apnoea/hypopnea syndrome. Thorax 1995;50:883–6.

51. Montplaisir J, Michaud M, Denesle R, et al. Periodic leg movements are not more prevalent in insomnia or hypersomnia but are specifically associated with sleep disorders involving a dopaminergic impairment. Sleep Med 2000;1:163–7.

52. Mahowald MW. Assessment of periodic leg movements is not an essential component of an overnight sleep study. Am J Respir Crit Care Med 2001;164: 1339–42.

53. Chervin RD. Periodic leg movements and sleepiness in patients evaluated for sleep-disordered breathing. Am J Respir Crit Care Med 2001;164:1454–8.

54. Chervin RD, Murman DL, Malow BA, et al. Cost-utility of three approaches to the diagnosis of sleep apnea: polysomnography, home testing, and empirical therapy. Ann Intern Med 1999;130:496–505.

55. Deutsch PA, Simmons MS, Wallace JM. Cost-effectiveness of split-night polysomnography and home studies in the evaluation of obstructive sleep apnea syndrome. J Clin Sleep Med 2006;2(2):145–53.

56. Ayas NT, Fox J, Epstein L, et al. Initial use of portable monitoring versus polysomnography to confirm obstructive sleep apnea in symptomatic patients: an economic decision model. Sleep Med 2010;11: 320–4.

57. White DP, Gibb TJ, Wall JM, et al. Assessment of accuracy and analysis time of a novel device to monitor sleep and breathing in the home. Sleep 1995;18(2):115–26.

58. Fletcher EC, Stich J, Yang KL. Unattended home diagnosis and treatment of obstructive sleep apnea without polysomnography. Arch Fam Med 2000;9: 168–74.

59. Golpe R, Jimenez A, Carpizo R. Home sleep studies in the assessment of sleep apnea/hypopnea syndrome. Chest 2002;122(4):1156–61.

Index

Note: Page numbers of article titles are in **boldface** type.

Sleep Med Clin 6 (2011) 387–391
doi:10.1016/S1556-407X(11)00075-0
1556-407X/11/$ – see front matter © 2011 Elsevier Inc. All rights reserved.

Moving?

Make sure your subscription moves with you!

To notify us of your new address, find your **Clinics Account Number** (located on your mailing label above your name), and contact customer service at:

Email: journalscustomerservice-usa@elsevier.com

800-654-2452 (subscribers in the U.S. & Canada)
314-447-8871 (subscribers outside of the U.S. & Canada)

Fax number: 314-447-8029

Elsevier Health Sciences Division
Subscription Customer Service
3251 Riverport Lane
Maryland Heights, MO 63043

*To ensure uninterrupted delivery of your subscription, please notify us at least 4 weeks in advance of move.

Printed and bound by CPI Group (UK) Ltd, Croydon, CR0 4YY

03/10/2024

01040354-0006